A Toxic Brain
Revelations from a Health Journey

Sandra C. Strauss

with Dan Watts, MD

DYNAMIC OPTIONS, INC.

Disclaimer: The medical information in this book is provided as an educational resource only and is not intended to be used or relied upon for any diagnostic or treatment purposes. This information should not be used as a substitute for professional diagnosis and treatment.

The lifestyle interventions discussed in this book should not be used as a substitute for consultation with your healthcare provider. Do not engage in any therapy or treatment without consulting a medical professional.

It is intended to provide helpful and informative material on the subjects addressed in the book. It is sold with the understanding that the author and publisher are not engaged in rendering medical, health, psychological or any other kind of professional services in the book. If the reader requires personal medical, health, or other assistance or advice, they should consult with a competent professional.

Neither the publisher nor the author is engaged in rendering professional advice to the individual reader. The ideas, procedures, and suggestions contained in this book are not intended as a substitute for consulting with your physician. All matters regarding your health require medical supervision.

The author and publisher specifically disclaim all responsibility for any liability, loss, or risk, personal or otherwise, that is incurred as a consequence, directly or indirectly, of the use and application of the contents of this book.

ISBN 978-1-66782-653-0

Dedication

This is dedicated to all who seek solutions for vibrant wellness, and to all practitioners integrating evolving science for optimizing patient health.

Praise for *A Toxic Brain—Revelations from a Health Journey*

"Over the past several years, it has become increasingly clear that Alzheimer's disease and Lewy body disease are multi-factorial, and the underlying drivers, such as specific toxins and pathogens, are beginning to be defined. *A Toxic Brain* is an important contribution to this evolving field, illustrating both the painstaking journey to ferret out the key disruptors of brain function for a patient, and the lessons learned—which could save many others in the future from similar fates. Author Sandra Strauss shows that she is at once a force of love and caring and of relentless biomedical pursuit."

Dale Bredesen, MD

Professor and author of *The New York Times* bestseller, *The End of Alzheimer's*

***

"The factors that need to align for optimal brain function are innumerable. But, as revealed in *A Toxic Brain*, many of the issues that threaten brain function today, and pose a risk for brain degeneration in the future, are now beginning to be delineated and validated. *A Toxic Brain* explores these myriad challenges and, more importantly, provides an empowering plan for both identifying these threats as well as defusing them. This is a solid action plan for brain health and resilience."

David Perlmutter, MD

Author, #1 *New York Times* bestseller, *Grain Brain*, and *Drop Acid*

***

"Sandra Strauss has taken a devastating journey, from the loss of her beloved husband to the failure of the conventional medical model to recognize environmental, infectious, and toxic causes of disease. She has transformed her grief into advocacy and hope for those and their families, facing unexplained mystery illnesses. Unfortunately, a journey I am all too familiar with but what led me to Functional Medicine where answers do exist!

"This book is a comprehensive overview of the many challenges seen with biotoxin exposures,and how to get to root causes and treatments, especially for neuro-psy-chiatric illnesses. This valuable tool not only provides resources for testing and knowledgeable practitioners, but also for the critical role of the care givers and support they need. It's a needed wake up call to help navigate the journey to whole-ness and healing with mind, heart, and spirit!"

Margaret Christensen, MD

CarpathiaCollaborative.com

Host, ToxicMoldproject.com

"I hope that this book finds its way into the hands of the growing number of people suffering with chronic complex illness. So many people are rejected and marginalized by our medical system in their search for health. This story gives voice to the journey of healing through functional medicine —an approach that validates the patient's experience of illness as real and legitimate. Many thanks for this empowering story!"

Anita Sadaty, MD
Redefining Health Medical

***

"*A Toxic Brain* offers valuable insights regarding the critical need for exploring the root causes underlying many of today's symptoms. It is an enlightening resource connecting toxins as a potent contributor to not only cognitive decline, but many other chronic illnesses impacting millions today. Helping my patients understand how these root causes play such a vital role in their own health destinies, is why this conversation is well-integrated into my practice."

Kate Wilson, DPT, PhD
The Lotus Center, Integral Healing & Wellness

***

"Through example and much study, this excellent book shares great insight into the many challenges we face with today's rampant toxic exposures and their impact upon our health. These are further compounded when seeking treatment for health issues in a medical system not adequately trained to address them. There is a critical need for the mainstream medical community, policy makers, and the public to recognize the indisputable connections between toxic exposures and health. With this wisdom and by adopting precision evaluation and treatment options, patient health will be greatly served."

Dick A. Chapman, DDS
Florida Integrative Dentistry

***

"This health journey is truly a riveting account and eye-opening read. It exemplifies important elements needed for proper evaluation and treatment of neurodegenerative issues, often overlooked in conventional medicine, that were only discovered through functional practices. *A Toxic Brain* offers readers an exhaustive review of medical and proven science-based strategies helpful in the prevention and treatment of toxic-related conditions. Sandra is a fierce advocate sharing insights in support of vibrant health destinies."

Kimberly Hartke
Publicist, Weston A. Price Foundation

Contents

Why I Wrote This Book

Without credible answers from mainstream medicine regarding what mysterious illness had stricken my robust and healthy husband Rick, I embarked upon a fervent journey of discovery. What had fired up so many strange symptoms that turned him into a stranger, seemingly overnight?

A team of specialists was unable to properly evaluate or treat his lingering and eventually fatal illness. It was a 12-year siege of ever-changing symptoms and cognition that—through traditional testing—defied diagnosis. Had it not been for one brilliant, resolute researcher who used revolutionary diagnostics for evaluation and treatment, the mystery of its cause may never have been solved. Rick died in 2016 from complications of an autoimmune, neurological condition triggered by toxicity, creating havoc in his body and brain.

Since most of Rick's doctors had rejected explanations of the actual causes, the exact nature of his illness would only be legitimized posthumously, with revelations stemming from research. I am compelled to provide the details of what I witnessed, documented, and learned from his illness, both inside and outside of mainstream medicine, in service to others.

Now in the third decade of the 21st century, many conventionally trained doctors have yet to embrace the evolving science of functional medicine that recognizes, evaluates, and treats patients with "a systems biology-based approach to patient care."[1] This approach focuses on identifying and addressing the root cause of disease. I share background on how some of these revolutionary insights and tools are transforming the health of patients, including conditions commonly viewed as irreversible. When millions are suffering and dying from autoimmune and neurological issues, it is time to shift the paradigm!

As a consumer educator with decades devoted to promoting strategies for wellness and well-being, I feel obligated to "unpack" my husband's case with all its complexities. The complicated nature of his neurological condition robbed our family of every shred of the familiar. As an endurance run of body, mind, and heart, I am also sharing the raw details of other matters related to Rick's illness—relationship rifts and shifts, family dynamics, care issues, legal consequences, and support strategies—in the hopes that it may help others navigate through their challenges.

If you or a loved one is suffering from a collection of symptoms impacting both body and brain, undergoing test after test in hopes of a diagnosis, or have been given one that does not seem to fit, read on. I wrote this book because answers do exist!

Introduction

In my role as the staunchest patient advocate for my late husband, Rick, I desperately wanted to know what suddenly transformed my healthy, 59-year-old husband into a debilitated stranger whom I barely recognized.

After reading "The Terrorist Inside My Husband's Brain" by Susan Schneider, the widow of Robin Williams—America's beloved actor-comedian—I experienced a visceral call to action. Although the initial news reports listed Williams' 2014 death as a suicide, it was later revealed that he had suffered from Lewy body dementia (LBD), a key factor in his self-inflicted demise. This progressive, debilitating neurological condition does indeed wreak terror on the body and brain, as we learned from Rick's own hellacious experience. In addition, the disease sparks suicidal thoughts. As a result, two beautiful spirits' lives were decimated by neurological nightmares.

In my quest for more answers, new information was revealed only while researching and writing this book. It further confirmed the toxic roots of Rick's illness. Science has now demonstrated the connections of toxicity with another dreaded neurological disease, a sub-type of Alzheimer's, and its possible connection to LBD. Yet, these toxic roots are now linked to many other chronic and life-threatening illnesses—autoimmune illnesses, cancers, heart disease, diabetes, to name a few.

Toxins are ubiquitous in today's inflammatory times. We're inhaling, ingesting and absorbing them often without the recognition of their impact upon our health. As science continues to confirm the relationship of symptoms and diseases to toxicity, it serves as a wake up call for us all.

It was an eerie realization reminiscent of an episode from *The Twilight Zone*, Rod Serling's classic 1950s and '60s television series featuring freakish science fiction and suspense stories. Could there be legions of people suffering from inflamed bodies and brains, with the roots of their illnesses not being identified early enough? Or treated with therapies that might possibly change their health destinies? These questions begged for confirmation.

The much-loved Williams had yet another role to play: spotlighting this more unfamiliar neurodegenerative condition, which was not as well recognized a few years ago.

Rick had always been blessed with robust health, a brilliant brain, and a fulfilling career of service, all enveloped within a happy 27-year-long marriage and loving family. Seemingly overnight, he became acutely ill with a multitude of symptoms—bizarre changes in personality and behavior accompanied by tremors, a bloody rash, wrenching gut and head pain, photosensitivity, and abdominal jerking, and many others.

While I first believed all these symptoms appeared overnight, I now understand that really was not the case at all. His body was a silent, ticking time bomb, and when a multitude of symptoms became apparent, this instantly transformed our realities and our destinies. Something did not just hit him "out of the blue." Yet, Rick rarely consulted with a doctor or shared his health concerns with me. Now, he was no longer able to conceal what he desperately had to have been hiding: something horrible had happened to his brain. There was no question about it. I was scared what this all meant.

While inflammation fired up Rick's neurological nightmare, none of his conventional evaluations addressed these triggers. Mainstream medicine typically focuses on the diagnosing of diseases and the treatment of symptoms, usually prescribing drugs or surgery, rather than finding the imbalances in the body that may be causing them. Rick's case serves as a quintessential example of how multiple inflammatory agents launched a cascade of imbalances that were never properly evaluated or treated by conventional medicine.

Even years after my husband was stricken, the underlying causes of these neurodegenerative and other chronic maladies, and the diagnostic testing available to evaluate and treat them, are not being recognized or adopted fast enough by mainstream healthcare practitioners. We cannot afford to wait! This tsunami is devastating lives and swamping precious resources. In "Tip of the Iceberg," a 2019 paper for the National Institute of Health's Institute on Aging, a group of doctors said between 2010-15 Alzheimer's and related dementia global costs rose 35%, to $818 billion (US) and could hit $2 trillion by 2030.[1] That doesn't include the collateral damage it causes to caregivers.

Now, after Rick's death, I am sharing details of his undignified and frightening fall from seemingly perfect health, including the roller coaster ride of my own emotional highs and lows. I offer our experience, including personal details about Rick's sometimes wild, uncharacteristic behavior and personality changes, for anyone who might be facing a similar situation and wondering what happened to their loved one.

In my role as witness, scribe, and educator, I have compiled the details of our family's journey to provide background for:

- Patients and their loved ones, who may be experiencing a similarly confusing, frustrating journey in search of answers.

- Health practitioners, to encourage adopting functional evaluation methods to discover underlying organic reasons driving patient symptoms and the therapies and lifestyle interventions needed to correct them. For those who have patients with brain or behavioral issues, to consider neurotoxicity, Chronic Inflammatory Response Syndrome (CIRS), toxic encephalopathy, Lewy body dementia,

Alzheimer's Type-3 (toxic-related), and autoimmune disorders as underlying conditions.

- Industry leaders and government regulators, to recognize how both production and manufacturing of products and regulations regarding them can either support the health, safety, and protection of our citizens, or have the potential to create and sustain chronic health issues.

- Readers interested in learning more about supporting their own brain health by understanding the root causes leading to neurological inflammation, common symptoms and behaviors associated with it, lifestyle interventions to help prevent its occurrence, and strategies for managing life when the unexpected strikes.

For the most part, Rick's mainstream medical teams were compassionate and caring. Yet they were not trained to look holistically, so they mainly focused on Rick's brain and behavioral issues. All the other physical symptoms he experienced were signs a functional practitioner would have noticed, inquired about, or tested for. His evaluation in conventional practices included plenty of imaging studies but could not reveal all the biochemical reactions causing his symptoms to flare. I include information about functional evaluation and some of their therapies later in the book.

In presenting Rick's case history, I have drawn from an extensive compilation of my own detailed observations of his changing symptoms and behavior, the treatments that appeared to work, and the ones that did not. I have highlighted some of the email exchanges with practitioners chronicling Rick's lab reports, neuropsychological testing results, medications he was prescribed, and other support documents gathered throughout his illness.

As a man whose career was dedicated to serving others, Rick loved the concept of "pay it forward," inspired by the movie of the same name. This book is his legacy—to pay it forward, so others might benefit from the pieces of the neurological puzzle that took years for us to assemble and is now being continually reaffirmed by practitioners of advanced medicine.

***

This is a fitting place to introduce Dan Watts, MD, a quadruple-board certified physician with decades of experience in both conventional and functional disciplines. He is the founder and director of The Renewal Point in Sarasota, Florida, focused on both prevention and transforming health through integrative assessments and therapies.

Upon relocating to Florida in 2018 while seeking a functional practitioner for my own healthcare, I was referred to Dr. Watts, who is known for his stellar reputation and an impressive list of credentials. We first met during his presentation highlighting the impact of toxins upon health. What a welcome discovery—a doctor who understood toxicity and other root causes of health issues! He immediately won my confidence and trust.

Later, as his patient, I shared with him that I was writing a book recounting Rick's toxic-related illness and revelations learned from that journey. He graciously offered to review it and I'm grateful for his wisdom and guidance in creating this resource for today's toxic times.

Life presents us with opportunities that often serve to shift the direction of our lives. Dr. Watts shares his inspiration for the paradigm shift in his own medical practice, his battle and that of his wife from toxic-related illnesses, his passion for getting to the root cause of health issues, and other insights as a functional/integrative physician.[2]

An Eye-Opening Perspective for Transforming Patient Care

More than twenty years ago my mother-in-law, Fannie Belle Burnett, was diagnosed by a neurologist with Parkinson's disease, exhibiting pill rolling tremor, postural changes, slower movement, cognitive impairment, rigid muscles, and other Parkinsonian-related symptoms. Although she was being treated with medication, her symptoms progressively worsened over the next two years. Parkinsonian groups were woefully pessimistic: "Just wait until it gets worse, Fannie Belle; then you can get an electric wheelchair."

Well, my strong-willed mother-in-law wanted nothing to do with going downhill without a fight! She explored other avenues and sought the wisdom offered in the emerging field of functional medicine.

One doctor in particular, Dr. David Perlmutter in Naples, Florida, was successfully treating Parkinson's patients. Under Dr. Perlmutter's care, not only did her symptoms improve dramatically over the next two years, but his treatment enhanced her quality of life in so many ways. Fannie Belle miraculously improved through the wisdom of integrative/functional medicine.

When she later returned to her neurologist in Memphis, Tennessee, her doctor was so impressed with her progress, he remarked, "Fannie Belle, you are doing so much better with the medication we last gave you."

"Why doctor, I've been off all the medication for over a year, and I feel great!" she replied.

Indeed, my mother-in-law's experience spared her the usual fate of Parkinson's patients, leading to a near Parkinson's-symptom-free life. Watching her miraculous recovery served as my own inspiration for transforming my practice into one based upon integrative and functional medicine.

Now, with more than two decades dedicated to integrative medicine, our medical team has assisted hundreds of patients in looking and feeling their best through proactive, preventative, and regenerative measures available through functional evaluations and therapies.

Dan Watts, MD

***

There are so many details to share in this neurological journey it is not possible to relate all of them. I am especially sharing the ones that were overlooked or dismissed so you might be inspired to explore them. Rick's underlying issues were not properly addressed by his traditional healthcare practitioners, who focused primarily on treating his symptoms with medications, rather than exploring what was causing them. Yet, it was precisely by identifying what had caused his symptoms that would ultimately reveal answers.

Rather than relating the details of these root causes in describing the journey of his illness, more information regarding their significance is provided in subsequent sections, as well as the tools and technologies which are transforming health destinies. For your convenience, a glossary is provided in the back for definitions of acronyms, medical terminology, and other terms featured.

Lastly, entwined within a debilitating, neurological illness, the need for caregiving must be addressed. The final chapters feature the challenges I encountered as a caregiver with its heartaches and lessons for the heart, along with strategies and proactive measures that can be taken in preparation.

Navigating the unknown with an open mind and open heart reveal miraculous discoveries for the body, mind, and spirit.

Sandra Strauss

For more about her role as a champion of wellness and vibrant aging, visit:
SandraStrauss.com.

Part 1

Our Personal Journey

Chapter 1
The Way We Were

Before the Cascade of Symptoms

As a vocational rehabilitation counselor, Rick's passion was helping the disabled—working on behalf of those whose lives and livelihoods had been impacted by an accident, a chronic illness, someone's negligence, or by a permanent brain injury. He also served as an expert witness, establishing a litigation consulting practice and testifying in cases that included vaccine injuries, toxic worksites, and traumatic brain injuries. Attorneys hired him for his expertise to assess wage loss and recommend the requirements of ongoing care for legal settlements.

Rick was a devoted husband and involved father, loved for his wit, wisdom, and big heart. He was a man of integrity with a stellar reputation. He was my rock for more than 30 years, totally grounded in all the right stuff. In fact, a local bakery must have known too, because on his 50th birthday cake, they inscribed, "Happy Birthday, Rock!"

From our first date in 1972, his love of positive psychology was one of the things that attracted me to him. His first gift to me was the book, *I Am Lovable and Capable*, by Sid Simon, a prolific author on values, self-esteem, and subjects closest to the heart. That set the tone for our relationship. We were on the same page, affirming the best and highest in one another. Indeed, Rick was a master of affirmation. He uplifted us with his words and affirmed the best in me and our two daughters by encouraging us to pursue our goals, cheering us on to achieve them, and then finding ways to celebrate our accomplishments. He truly embodied unconditional love, and I was especially grateful for our mutually supportive marriage.

Dancing in a Dream Life

Summer 2003

With his career as a vocational rehabilitation consultant, Rick was constantly juggling a heavy caseload of clients. During his weeks away that summer, while working on a class action suit in the Arctic region of Canada, we eagerly anticipated our family adventures together.

Rick and I enjoyed creating unforgettable memories for our family and relished every chance to rev up our adventurous souls somewhere beyond the familiar. We knew our regular family escapades would soon be nearing an end since our oldest daughter, Stephanie, was now a junior in college and Stacy was entering her senior year in high school.

A picture of a Bavarian castle, its majestic spires rising into the blue sky, hung on our refrigerator. Amid the daily bustle of our household, as well as looming work deadlines, the picture of that magic castle became a touchstone for me, a faraway place that beckoned my soul reminding me that a well-deserved rest was just a flight away.

A year later, as we were waltzing across the dance floor in Vienna, Austria, I was having one of those "Please, pinch me if this is real!" moments. Rick and I and our two daughters had just visited the Bavarian castle, Neuschwanstein (the inspiration for Disneyland's Sleeping Beauty Castle), perched magnificently atop the Austrian Alps. This was my long-envisioned dream come to life. Indeed, the Strauss family was smack dab in the middle of a fairytale vacation, dancing to the music of a Strauss waltz, composed by my husband's namesake—a much more famous Richard Strauss.

While enjoying the breathtaking splendor of Bavaria and beyond, Rick and I began plotting more travel adventures as soon-to-be empty nesters. Costa Rica was calling me next with its lush landscapes, zip-wire adventures, and tropical rainforests. When we returned from Bavaria, we posted a new touchstone picture of cascading waterfalls surrounded by exotic flowers on our refrigerator: our next escape into paradise.

But it was not to be.

Chapter 2
Awakening to a New Reality

March 2004

Just six months later, those dreams of paradise were dashed when the unexpected suddenly turned our family upside down, bringing life as we knew it to a halt. One early March morning, I awoke to find Rick slumped over his computer. The screen displayed the same page it had when I kissed him goodnight the evening before. Rick was a workaholic with a sharp, analytical mind and a reputation for coming up with award-winning solutions, so I thought he had just burned the midnight oil to complete a client report. But this was not his usual style—he was not acting at all like himself.

Usually, nothing rattled Rick. His calm demeanor and rational ways had always been a perfect complement to my capriciousness. But now, he was visibly shaken. His hands trembled. He confessed that his steel-trap brain hadn't been working in the same way for some time. I recalled a very strange, penetrating gaze he had flashed me the evening before and had wondered what that was all about.

Later, I'd recall that Rick had made a few rather uncharacteristic and unusual comments lately, which I had chalked up to his increasing withdrawal into his office. My attempts to inquire, "What's wrong?" did not reveal any insights. I presumed it was from stress, or perhaps a very silent, midlife crisis was making him especially introspective. Whatever it was, it felt eerily abnormal.

Now I recognized: something was horribly wrong. Rick was well-known in legal circles for his brilliant work. His gifts of research and assessment had built a highly specialized career as he helped clients economically rebuild their lives following loss or illness. The legal system is very demanding; timeliness and accuracy are critical. Over the years, Rick had accumulated a thick file of attorney correspondence attesting to his expertise, and he was in high demand as an expert witness.

His brain had never failed him before, at least not that I had noticed. But upon further reflection, I recognized that Rick had said and done some rather weird things over the last few weeks. Client reports were strewn in piles around his office, waiting to be completed. He admitted he could not process all the information swirling around in his brain. Now he repeatedly echoed the same phrase: "I'm leaving you with nothing." I had no idea if he had just wiped out our savings or what else might have triggered that comment. All I knew was that I woke up to a new reality.

The Search for Answers Begins

I no longer recognized the man I once knew completely. The man I had always counted on, who was so dependable, and who cherished me, totally morphed into a stranger, stricken by something that stole away his very essence.

For the first 27 years of our marriage, Rick was rarely ever sick. Now, I was filled with both fear and confusion. Beyond his inability to focus and concentrate, he had tremors and weird, undulating, abdominal thrusts. His back, chest, and arms were covered in an oozy, bloody rash. He had difficulty keeping his eyes open, and he was moving slowly and strangely.

Shortly after that March morning wake-up call, I scheduled an appointment with Rick's internist. His doctor had conducted a full exam on him just six months before and knew Rick as a healthy patient. He advised a psychiatric consult and I immediately called to schedule an appointment, but everyone was either booked, some up to several months, or was not taking new patients. I finally booked an appointment with "Dr. G.," a psychiatrist in McLean, Virginia, just a few days later.

On the way to the doctor's office, going 60 miles per hour on the Washington, DC beltway, Rick kept putting his hand on the door handle, as if wanting to jump out. Driving alone with him, I felt terrified and helpless. He cast me a devilish grin, saying, "Don't worry, I won't jump." That wasn't the least bit reassuring. I didn't recognize this stranger riding next to me.

After his consultation, Dr. G. suggested that Rick should be admitted to the psychiatric ward at Virginia Hospital Center in Arlington for a thorough evaluation. Admittedly, while I understood the need, it was still surreal. My husband's behavior was so totally uncharacteristic of him. I was hopeful their medical team would discover the cause of the problem from the multitude of tests conducted, which would include brain MRIs, blood work, CT scans, psychiatric evaluations, and more. However, they released Rick a week later without a definitive diagnosis. His hospital discharge papers only listed a suspected "generalized anxiety disorder." This seemed far more severe than an episode of anxiety.

Because Rick was a conscientious workaholic, psychiatrists initially suspected that he was suffering from a severe case of anxiety and depression caused by stress. That observation didn't seem to fit the Rick I knew—nothing ever seemed to rattle him. However, he was exhibiting behaviors I had never witnessed, and stress was likely at least one of the factors.

Back at home, the landscape of our lives was now definitely different. Rick didn't act or talk at all like the man I had long known. What was at the root of all his physical symptoms and such foreign behavior? I was confused and concerned by the realities that appeared daily, sometimes changing moment-by-moment.

Often, I observed him walking halfway up our stairs, then stopping and hanging over the banister. He collapsed occasionally, blacked out, and then couldn't remember what had happened. Sometimes he could barely speak, while other times he couldn't stop talking, releasing a string of almost inaudible words.

I kept encouraging Rick with positive affirmations and was shocked at his difficulty with repeating "I" statements. We had raised both our daughters on a steady diet of affirmations. Whatever was wrong, it had also robbed him of his personality and his well-known wit.

And why did Rick have such a hard time keeping his eyes open? The response from the hospital psychiatrist had been, "Maybe he doesn't want to be here (meaning in this world)." That idea did not fit the Rick I knew—a proud, loving family man who often shared his family photos with clients. I couldn't give the doctor's speculative response any credence. After all, he was viewing Rick through the eyes of a psychiatrist. Later, I discovered that Rick was photosensitive, another symptom of toxicity, and light strained his eyes.

Rick's behavior became more bizarre as his symptoms escalated. He often stayed in his home office with the door shut. More than once I heard him talking to himself and muffling occasional screams. Sometimes, I heard him carrying on a conversation with no one around. *This wasn't a case of anxiety.* I became convinced that Rick was suffering from something so rare that we were unable to get an accurate diagnosis or treatments that worked.

Rick's strange behavior without confirmation from all his testing, led his neurologist to believe his illness was psychiatric in nature. Months later, Dr. G. dropped the "D" word—"dementia"—as a possibility. How could Rick have dementia? He was only 59 and that seemed way too young. Plus, the full spectrum of his symptoms was totally uncharacteristic of Alzheimer's, as understood by me and numerous neurologists who had consulted on his case.

Rick continually aced repeated mini mental tests, then the standard tool for dementia assessment. He always correctly answered the usual questions of "What day is it? What season is it? Who's the president?" Dr. G. asked him to draw a clock and although his drawing skills had never been very good, it appeared he passed that, too. Yet, his brain clearly wasn't functioning. After all, Rick was a highly intelligent guy who was well-acquainted with those tests from his own career, working with doctors and reviewing clients' medical histories. Was he drawing upon his professional background in diagnostic evaluation to fake these tests?

Unfortunately, before Dr. G. was able to conduct more tests, he died of heart issues, and his office closed. We lost a vital connection to a trusted, empathetic doctor who was open to exploring possible organic reasons underlying Rick's illness.

Subsequent consultations with several neurologists suggested Parkinson's disease. Other diagnoses considered were Creutzfeldt-Jakob disease, a rare, fast degenerative, fatal brain disorder; and stiff person syndrome (SPS), a rare autoimmune disease affecting the nervous system, specifically the brain and spinal cord. I couldn't understand why conventional medicine with all their diagnostic tests couldn't piece together the symptoms Rick was experiencing.

For more than a year after the onset of Rick's symptoms, we sought consultations with health practitioners from both conventional and integrative practices. Conventional doctors viewed only the symptoms associated with their own expertise or specialty, without considering the multiple health issues Rick was experiencing. Worse yet, none of the drugs they prescribed helped to relieve Rick's pain or resolve his symptoms.

Several trusted friends recommended we consult with a naturopath/acupuncturist in Bethesda. This was our first foray into natural medicine; the practitioner's reputation and patient chairside manner, as well as the innovative technology she used for Rick's evaluation, gained my trust immediately.

She prescribed Rick enzymes, homeopathy tinctures for thyroid, adrenal support, and nutrition supplements—including minerals, vitamin B complex, and vitamin C. I was hopeful that by combining both conventional and natural medicine, his health would be restored. However, as time went on, my optimism dimmed.

While the holistic health professionals identified issues linked to heavy metals, biotoxins, and resulting imbalances, their homeopathic remedies didn't seem to be creating any noticeable improvement in Rick's condition. Admittedly, perhaps I had set my own expectations too high. I was convinced that by doing everything both mainstream and holistic practitioners recommended, Rick's health would improve. However, months went by and nothing changed.

Mounting Concerns

Prior to Rick's illness, we were the ultimate multi-tasking team. Rick took care of all those time-consuming, pesky, ever-present financial details of life that I didn't like to do—taxes, investigating insurance plans, getting the girls' tuition plans squared away for college, monitoring investments, and paying bills.

Right before Rick lost his executive functioning ability, we were in the process of refinancing our home and tax season was looming. Rick had been my personal GPS system—managing and locating data was his gift. Now I was on my own, searching and scrambling for documents. I regretted I hadn't paid more attention to financial matters over the years. I had taken for granted that Rick would always take care of the stuff I hated to do. Now I had no choice; it was all my responsibility. I became the paperwork priestess and the detail diva, roles which were not my forte.

But now the paperwork had multiplied beyond what he had ever managed. Every day papers piled up from his business, my business, and our personal lives. Plus, I had to devote more time to deciphering the gobbledygook of medical forms and insurance policies associated with his illness.

We were running up huge medical costs that required constant monitoring and nonstop insurance bills that required the same. I was overwhelmed with all of this, as well as caring for my almost 90-year-old mother, who was in the throes of her own dementia and cancer treatment.

I had to create a new dance of rearranging competing priorities. My days were often focused on tending to the countless details. Additionally, beyond all the time-consuming tasks and Rick's endless stream of medical tests and appointments, I now served as the sole parent. I did my best to be an emotional anchor for our two girls, who wondered where their dad had gone and if he would ever return.

Now, life was spinning out needs simultaneously in almost every arena of life—physical, mental, financial, emotional, and spiritual. Our relationship and roles transformed. Care issues surfaced, and constant stress was taking a devastating toll on our family's well-being. Even with all the support from people who uplifted my spirits and provided guidance, I was overwhelmed with all the details demanding my time and concentration.

Our combined livelihood was also in jeopardy. As attorneys called to inquire about Rick's availability as a consultant, I optimistically joked, a la *Terminator* style: "He's the Strauss-anator! He'll be back!" A few months later, I could no longer postpone the inevitable and began turning away Rick's business, referring cases—coincidentally, many toxic tort cases—to his colleagues. Ultimately, I would need to close his consulting business. Meanwhile I was trying to keep my own business of professional speaking, writing, and public relations afloat. I longed for the good old days in every way.

In April 2004, Stacy, our then high school senior, wanted me to attend a weekend retreat with her at a regional retreat center on Maryland's Eastern Shore. Parents were invited to witness a special ceremony that weekend for graduating seniors. I was only able to go to the retreat because of the kindness of true friends Brenda, Lowell, Paige, and Tony, who volunteered shifts for Rick's round-the-clock care.

Although I had planned to ride with Stacy on the church bus, care arrangements for Rick collapsed at the last minute due to his strange behavior the night before. When I went to bed that evening, Rick was sprawled on our stairs, looking at a map of Maryland and repeatedly saying, "You'll never get there! You'll never get there!" He kept drawing circles over and over on the map, afraid I'd never get across the Chesapeake Bridge. I assured him I'd be fine, but this was freaking me out. He refused my offers of help to get him into bed.

The next morning, I found Rick in the same position, still on the stairs and drawing circles on the map as he expressed the same concerns. With his hallucinations, it was hard to know where his mind had gone. I was torn. In front of me was a stranger in obvious mental distress, yet Stacy was already at the church retreat. Especially now, with our family life in such turmoil, I wanted to be with her as a much-needed grounding force.

I called Brenda to tell her about Rick's condition and told her I was conflicted as to what to do. Knowing what the last six weeks had been for us, she insisted that I go to the retreat. I was beyond grateful to see Brenda's smiling face first thing that Saturday morning. Rick and I had shared a long friendship with Brenda and her husband, Bob, and we were richly blessed that they would (and did) do to help us throughout Rick's illness. Brenda was giving me the greatest gift: a slice of time to spend with Stacy, albeit with an illusion of normalcy at the church retreat-and-graduation ceremony.

After I crossed the Chesapeake Bridge, more than halfway to the retreat center, Brenda called, saying Rick was manic. I put in an emergency call to his psychiatrist. Suspecting he might have encephalitis, the doctor said Rick needed to go to the emergency room immediately. Brenda urged me to continue to the retreat and promised that she would take him to the hospital. Because of her insistence, I agreed.

By the time a doctor saw Rick at the ER, his mania had subsided. Since Rick's demeaner seemed perfectly normal, the physician wondered why Rick was even there. This scenario of strange behavior, followed by the nearly normal, would repeat itself on many occasions. It caused both anger and confusion in me and all who witnessed it, because it made us look like the crazy ones. Plus, we were not getting any answers.

By now, I was exhausted from the constant siege of Rick's bizarre behavior, and still waiting for a definite diagnosis of what was causing it all. Every day something new seemed to arise. I documented everything for clues, in hopes one doctor, or a medical team, could piece it all together.

Imagine the frustration our family endured, never knowing what to expect. The girls were embarrassed by their dad's very weird behavior, and I kept praying for guidance to sustain my spirit throughout the daily chaos. Suspended in a world without answers, we wondered, worried, and waited, struggling to find hope within our heartaches.

Daycare Respite

May 2004

Fortunately, we had a supportive social network. Help poured forth. Maureen, a recently retired social worker, recommended Rick be placed in an adult daycare program. Several months after his illness struck, I realized that Rick was not going to return to work anytime soon and I needed to put my energy into generating income as well as some relief from being a full-time caregiver.

As a consultant, I did not have the benefit of any family leave time. The closest senior center was 30 minutes away without traffic and 60 minutes during rush hour. A team of loving spirits from our church volunteered to drive him to the center while the county transportation service brought him home. Some days he could not go because he was too exhausted or symptomatic. Other days he would basically sit in a chair, unwilling or unable to do much else.

It became apparent early on that Rick's case was not being viewed holistically. It was all too reminiscent of the legendary Indian parable about the blind men and an elephant. You likely know the story of six blind travelers, with each one creating their own version of reality from a limited perspective and experience. Likewise, different doctors with their own specialty filtered my husband's symptoms through that specific lens of their experience. Each ordered tests and prescribed an ever-changing array of chemical cocktails in hopes of discovering something or a combination that would work to address his diverse symptoms.

However, they didn't address the root causes—his body's unfortunate genetics, triggered by long-term toxic exposures from chemicals, toxic metals, biotoxins, infections, gut issues, and others. We would discover this later.

Chapter 3
Seasons of Despair

June 2004

By early June 2004, Rick had undergone a series of traditional tests, ranging from MRIs and lumbar punctures (spinal taps) to electroencephalograms (EEG) and CT scans without any indication of a problem. Desperately needing answers, we eagerly looked forward to learning more from Rick's forthcoming hospitalization at the world-renowned Johns Hopkins Hospital in Baltimore, Maryland.

When it came time to drive to Johns Hopkins, Rick started acting wild and refused to get into the car. Our then18-year-old daughter, Stacy, and I had no choice but to stuff him into the backseat, kicking and screaming. Stacy jumped in after him and tried to calm him to no avail.

After driving about two miles from our home with Rick screaming and out of control, I knew it would be impossible to safely drive him to the hospital, at least two hours away in heavy commuter traffic. Fortunately, I spied a police cruiser and pulled over. The officer called an ambulance, which arrived within minutes to take us to Fairfax Inova Hospital in Falls Church, Virginia.

From the front seat of the ambulance with sirens blaring, I called our minister, who was well-aware of Rick's ever-changing behavior. She agreed to meet us at the emergency room (we definitely needed plenty of prayer support!) After doing a quick assessment in the ER, a doctor said he could be released. What??!!

Afraid to continue the drive to Baltimore since I envisioned more of the same while ensnared in traffic on the Capital Beltway, I called again upon my friend, Brenda. Having witnessed Rick's aberrant behavior while caring for him two months earlier, she volunteered to drive us to Johns Hopkins. Before leaving the ER, I asked that Rick be sedated so we could safely travel. Fortunately, we arrived without incident.

Upon admission, Rick underwent his umpteenth mini mental test and again passed it with flying colors. Brenda and I looked at each other in disbelief. How was it possible that he could be so cognizant and then moments later exhibit such bizarre behavior? We both had become suspicious he was "playing" us.

I met with his team at the hospital and provided background of his long-term, chemical exposures and a detailed account of his symptoms. I returned home that evening confident this prestigious medical center would put the puzzling picture together. However, unbeknownst to me, Rick refused a repeat of the spinal tap he had had just two months earlier. Without notifying me first, the hospital discharged him two days later without the full benefit of evaluation from the Hopkins' staff.

Because of Rick's refusal we missed our opportunity for what we hoped would be a definitive diagnosis. Instead, the hospital released him with a diagnosis of major depression and possible dementia, with a suspicion of Hashimoto encephalopathy (a rare disorder characterized by impaired brain function). Blood work showed he was ANA (antinuclear antibody) positive, indicating autoimmune issues, although I didn't fully understand those ramifications at the time. I did not have the opportunity to discuss the diagnoses with his treating clinicians and was unable to reinstate his admission for continuing evaluation. The summary of his discharge report:

Neurology report impression: The acute onset and rapid progression of symptoms in a middle-aged man with no previous psychiatric history suggest an underlying neurological cause for the depressive symptoms. Hashimoto's encephalopathy, prion (note: a rare neurodegenerative disorder), paraneoplastic disease (a rare disorder triggered by an abnormal immune system), and other rapid progressive dementias were considered.

"**Hashimoto encephalopathy** (HE) is a condition characterized by onset of confusion with altered level of consciousness; seizures; and jerking of muscles (myoclonus). Psychosis, including visual hallucinations and paranoid delusions, has also been reported. The exact cause of HE is not known but may involve an autoimmune or inflammatory abnormality. It is associated with Hashimoto's thyroiditis, but the nature of the relationship between the two conditions is unclear. Most people with HE respond well to corticosteroid therapy or other immunosuppressive therapies, and symptoms typically improve or resolve over a few months."[1]

The symptoms of Hashimoto encephalopathy can vary from person to person. They most often include sudden or subacute onset of confusion with alteration of consciousness. Some people have multiple, recurrent episodes of neurological deficits with cognitive dysfunction. Others experience a more progressive course characterized by slowly progressive cognitive impairment with dementia, confusion, hallucinations, or sleepiness. In some cases, rapid deterioration to coma can occur.

In addition to confusion and mental status changes, symptoms may include seizures and myoclonus (muscle jerking) or tremor. Psychosis, including visual hallucinations and paranoid delusions, has also been reported.

When thyroid antibodies interact with brain antibodies, it can result in Thyroiditis encephalopathy or Hashimoto encephalopathy, with symptoms in alignment with those Rick was manifesting.

Although I didn't have Rick's lab results from that hospitalization, I did have a copy of Rick's bloodwork from the following February. It indicated his thyroid panel numbers were out of range, as were his red and white blood cell counts. The numbers stood out in boldface as out-of-range, so why were they ignored—especially with Hashimoto's encephalopathy so in alignment with Rick's symptoms? Unfortunately, at the time, I was unfamiliar with the connection of thyroid issues. Otherwise, I would have likely hounded doctors to further investigate.

My optimism vanished. Upon his release, I was once again frustrated by the lack of a definitive diagnosis. At home, his behavior continued to be bewildering and increasingly distressing.

A Time of Decline

June-August 2004

A few days following Rick's discharge from Johns Hopkins, Stacy graduated from high school. To maintain the now ever-elusive "status quo" in the Strauss household, I volunteered for helping at the senior all-night party, with my shift ending around 2:00 a.m. When I returned home, my older daughter, Stephanie, warned me that her dad was acting strangely again.

Shortly after I arrived home, Rick collapsed on the floor screaming, "My head's electric! My head's electric!" He thrashed and wailed in pain, with what appeared to be a seizure, accompanied by nearly non-stop screaming for about 45 minutes. Still without a confirmed diagnosis or resources, I was at a loss as to how to handle his increasingly confusing physical and behavioral issues.

Rick's health continued to deteriorate. He lived in a fog and our family in a nightmare without receiving an explanation that made any sense. Day after day, he suffered multiple symptoms and pain. We never knew what to expect or how long he would suffer without relief. His constantly changing symptoms varied in intensity and duration. They included crushing migraines, gripping stomach pain, joint pain, lightning bolt sensations, seizures, shortness of breath, wheezing, red eyes, light sensitivity, difficulty sleeping, fatigue, and nerve pain that he likened to being on fire. Once I learned that his body and brain were consumed by inflammation, it would all make sense.

From mid-June to September of 2004, I observed a wide range of symptoms and behaviors, which I shared with his treatment team.

> **Behavior:** In addition to his cognitive deficiencies and lack of focus, Rick's behavior has changed significantly towards his family and friends. He recognizes us and knows who we are, but he's become emotionally vacant—he doesn't hug any of us, strike up conversations, ask us many questions, or relate in any of the ways that once made him so lovable.

> Rick has become apathetic and negative. His characteristic warmth used to light up the lives of his family and friends, as well as strangers. Now, he doesn't make much of an effort to relate to anyone. He makes socially inappropriate comments, and I cannot predict how he will act when he is with others.

> Rick is also strangely fixated on never having enough food in the house, although two refrigerators are well-stocked and the pantry is full.

> **Language:** Most apparent is the change in Rick's language. He speaks in a soft, expressionless drone, often barely audible. When we ask him to repeat himself or speak louder, he says he cannot, which frustrates us.

> At other times, he speaks haltingly in gasp-like breaths, repeating a word or sentence several times, e.g., "The thing is ... the thing is ... " and then "jabbering" almost nonstop.

> Even around others, he does not try to engage in conversation. Instead, he spins out a string of observations (e.g., "It's raining," or "She's coming in the door," etc.) or thoughts not really intended for others to respond. He continues to ruminate.

> **Hygiene:** Rick's lost motivation to take showers. He does not like to wash his hair or brush his teeth.

> **Diet:** Rick had previously lost about 40 pounds, but he now seems to be foraging frequently and gaining weight back. He has a penchant for chocolate and sugar—I have found him eating sugar straight out of the canister or sucking on sugar cubes. (Reader note: Craving sugary foods is a noted sign of having candida/yeast issues with a potential risk for brain inflammation.)

Movement: Rick moves slowly and says he sometimes cannot move at all. He has told me that he blanks out at times. He also exhibits abdominal, undulating movements. Different parts of his body are constantly jerking as though he is experiencing jolts of electricity. Rick reports that he is physically weak. He is not comfortable in any position—sitting, standing, or laying down.

Rick has had a series of "convulsions," with his body writhing to the point I thought he would have a heart attack. The first episode lasted for about three hours, including 45 minutes of screaming; three days later, he had another that lasted about an hour. After each, his shirt was drenched in sweat. He said his brain was "electric" and he had severe headaches during and immediately following the episodes.

Eyes: He used to have good eye contact with people; now he rarely looks people in the eyes. Rick's eyes also seem to have a distant look and he has difficulty keeping them open.

Summary: Rick's behavior has changed dramatically in the last four months, which has taken a toll on our family—especially not knowing what is causing it. We are all extremely frustrated that a definite diagnosis has not been offered, with a corresponding treatment plan and prognosis. None of the many medications have offered relief of symptoms. We are hoping Rick can be hospitalized again to be properly evaluated and offered therapies that can better support his health.

I continue to search the Internet for answers. Rick exhibits all the classic symptoms associated with Lewy body dementia (LBD). Dr. G. and I had discussed this as a possibility in the past. As I see the condition progress, I am more certain it is.

While Alzheimer's disease is the most prevalent type of dementia, there are other types affecting different parts of the brain. It's still a mystery to me why none of his treating health professionals, including a number of neurologists with whom we consulted, never considered LBD! Eleven years later, after being poked, probed, and prodded by countless healthcare providers, Rick's last treating neurologist, pronounced that he was in the final stages of Lewy body dementia, as described in Appendix D: "Common Symptoms of Lewy Body Dementia."

Rick's neurologist, who had issued a thorough series of conventional tests for Rick and found nothing specific, referred us to the Memory Disorders Clinic at a Virginia hospital. Here are the main highlights from that August 24, 2004 evaluation:

Memory: Poor concentration and easily distractible. Difficulty describing elements of his personal and recent history, forgetful.

Cognition: Spontaneous speech revealed mild loosened thoughts, with rumination.

Impression: His neurologic examination is significant for a bizarre affect and social interactions, soliloquy, pedolalia (infantile speech), echolalia (repeating words), some forgetfulness, poor attention, and concrete abstractions.

In terms of his amnestic disorder, I think it is extremely likely this is due to a psychiatric condition. I agree that it is odd for such a problem to come on at this age. However, a very thorough and impressive workup has failed to find another likely explanation for his decline.

Non-psychiatric possibilities include stiff person syndrome in a man with odd affect and gait difficulties, primary or metastatic neoplastic or paraneoplastic disease, subacute infection, or possibly an atypical course of frontotemporal degeneration. (Note: this would later be revealed through additional testing.)

Functional and cognitive decline: I think that a psychiatric etiology is still the most likely and recommend electroconvulsive shock therapy. I think that it is time to face up to the strong and likely possibility that a psychiatric disorder is afoot. Finally, if he does have an atypical version of frontotemporal degeneration, there is no other further diagnostic work that I would suggest, except to follow him clinically and consider reimaging in 6-12 months.

Safety issues: He should not be left alone and should not be driving in his current state. Financial decisions and other legal matters should not be left in his sole hands.

Clearly, Mr. Strauss has represented a complex diagnostic situation. He and his wife are in a tough bind and are doing the best they can under trying circumstances. I certainly do hope that he gets definitive diagnostic and therapeutic care.

What a statement from a specialist who "hoped" that Rick would receive a definitive diagnosis! I was counting on this doctor to provide that hope!

A Temporary "Awakening"

Fall 2004

Month after month, neither doctors nor all the extensive medical tests they ordered, could offer any diagnosis. Some suspected dementia but discounted it because Rick's symptoms manifested differently from classic symptoms; others thought it was an uncharacteristic psychiatric manifestation. All they recommended were different combinations or strengths of antipsychotic, anti-convulsive or antidepressant drugs.

I continued to seek healing and answers beyond traditional medicine—acupuncture, acupressure, homeopathy, chelation IV drips, detox tablets, magnetic clay, essential oils, energy healings, prayer vigils, and more. Nothing was working.

One November afternoon, I received a phone call from the executive director at the adult daycare facility, who asked what I had been doing with Rick. "Everything I could!" I replied. She said keep it up because Rick had "awakened" that afternoon and was acting amazingly like a volunteer, not someone in need of support!

When I met Rick at the bus that evening, he was beaming a Cheshire cat grin. I called Lowell, Dotti, and a few other friends as witnesses. When we all gathered later that evening, with Rick witnessing such clarity, we all believed a miracle had taken place and he was on the road to full recovery.

However, it was short-lived. The next morning Rick told Joanna, one of his transportation team members: "I'm back in the fog." Indeed, just like that Rick had disappeared into it yet again. The despair we all felt reminded me of the question famed movie critic Roger Ebert made in his review of the 1990 movie, *Awakenings*: "If one has no hope, which is better: To remain hopeless, or to be given hope and then lose it again?"[2] Ironically, the film starred future LBD sufferer Robin Williams in the lead role of a doctor seeking answers to his patients' neurological issues.

Thanksgiving, 2004

The meds are not working. In fact, I wonder if it's of any value to continue them. I've been reviewing background about long-term effects, and I don't like what I'm reading.

Rick seems to be in a deeper fog than a few weeks ago. I try to keep him moving and engaged physically outside. It is pitiful to watch him rake leaves. He rakes a minute or so, then stops and talks to himself or just stands there, as if frozen in time. He also often repeats the same phrase, like "the History

Channel." Once, while I was choking in the kitchen, instead of responding to my distress, I heard him simply repeating, "The History Channel ... the History Channel."

While Rick can respond when spoken to, he is now barely audible. When our daughters were home for Thanksgiving, he barely spoke or showed any affection to them. This rips me up because they're trying so hard to love and understand him, but they're not getting anything in return.

Rick has no energy, no power, and the spirit of the man we have known and loved forever is now gone. If this continues into January, I will begin looking for alternative care. He's now entering the ninth month without any progress and there seems to be little more than I can do.

December 2004

In the middle of December, I hosted a 60th birthday bash for Rick, inviting many friends who had supported us and walked with us down the halls of darkness as they lighted our way. Rick was so sick he sat on the sofa, hunched over and out of it, trying to muster whatever energy he could to be the trouper he was at heart. I asked all to bring a candle to share their love and light.

My intention was to create a loving space, although Rick could not interact much. The candles were symbolic and burned bright, shining light during these darkest of days, reminding us of the Light that surrounds all circumstances.

Chapter 4
Continuing Concerns

January 2005

Another year, another email to Rick's treating neurologist updating her on his symptoms. I also shared his lab reports from integrative practitioners who had also evaluated Rick from their perspectives:

- Brain fog

- Jabbing abdominal pains, nausea

- Low body temperature, sometimes 94 or 95

- Cold and can't get warm

- Difficulty walking, moving

- Joint pain

- Blanking out

- Extreme fatigue

- Rash on back and chest noticed since onset

- Red eyes, but without pink eye stickiness

- Light sensitivity; can't keep eyes open

- Difficulty sleeping

- Anxiety

- Feels like skin crawling or jumping out of skin

- Tremors

- Difficulty speaking up

- Wheezing

I continued writing to Rick's conventionally trained neurologist, relating how—at the suggestion of a friend who suffered toxicity problems with symptoms like Rick's had subsequently reversed her condition through integrative medicine—we had also consulted with a medical doctor employing integrative therapies. From her earlier comments, I knew she did not support alternative therapies. However, from several heavy metals tests, Rick's results indicated high levels of lead, aluminum, cadmium, and others, and this may hold a link to his condition.

I added that an integrative doctor suspected Lyme disease. I mentioned to her that Rick had been tested back in the spring and although the blood test she requested was negative, we had learned that negative readings are not that uncommon, even though Lyme may be present. As a result, I told her, we had been treating Rick's condition with homeopathy, coupled with his prescribed medications, and would soon be consulting with his psychiatrist to review his current meds. Since Rick's second SPECT was evaluated as normal, we were not advised whether to continue the Namenda (prescribed by the neurologist to reduce mental confusion).

Here is a continuation of that email to his neurologist:

> "It has been a very frustrating, confusing time and I recognize that Rick's case has been perplexing. From information submitted to you earlier regarding the impact of Rick's long-term exposure to heavy metals—growing up on property which was eventually condemned by the EPA for toxic contamination—I believe this, coupled with the possibility of Lyme disease, are central to his case.

> Since his case is still unclear, I will not subject him to ECT which you've recommended. I am steadfast in my belief that the cause of his cognitive dysfunction and psychiatric disturbances is likely symptomatic of heavy metal toxins and Lyme, not psychiatrically based.

> I received an article today about Lyme disease stating that a patient may test negative for it, yet still be afflicted, especially if taking other medication. It can create many symptoms, mimicking Alzheimer's, ALS, irritable bowel syndrome (IBS), chronic fatigue, cognitive problems and many others and stated Lyme is often not recognized.

> Rick continues to have movement difficulties, joint pain, especially in his hips; fatigue, fluctuating body temperature ranging from 94 to 102 degrees, loss of executive function, cognitive difficulties, skin rashes, loss of appetite, flat affect, echolalia, nearly inaudible speech, and other symptoms.

> His poor health has been devastating to our family—emotionally, financially, and in every way imaginable. He was self-employed and because I'm also an independent consultant as well as his caregiver, I haven't been able to work much either.

> Rick has had more movement problems, difficulty in getting in and out of bed, walking, etc., causing increasing demands on my energy and time. I don't know what the future holds, but I need to begin investigating alternative care arrangements."

January 8

I provided Rick's treating psychiatrist with a New Year's update as well:

> "Rick is expressing more child-like behavior. I sometimes hear him whining in a child-like tone. He is also speaking gibberish, often repeating the same strange word or phrase.
>
> He moves very slowly and although I try to keep him active either outside or on the treadmill, it's only minutes before I find him back in bed or on the sofa.
>
> He continues to be emotionally numb, showing no concern or interest in either my daughters or me. His eyes are closed much of the time, and he has difficulty opening them when asked.
>
> I observe small muscle jerks or spasms, sometimes several times a minute, even while he's asleep. Earlier, I thought these may have been associated with his abdominal problems, but they seem to be a separate malady. He has lost his appetite and doesn't eat much.
>
> None of the medications seem to be working. I am concerned his brain has been infused with a chemical stew over the past year, so I really do not want to add anymore or try anything new, since nothing seems to be working. I am also afraid the mixture of meds may also be compounding some of his problems.
>
> I have enlisted the assistance of a senior care specialist to help me in determining care options. Rick has not been well enough to attend daycare except for two days during December."

Whispers of Desperation

After New Year's, the girls and I noticed that Rick became fascinated with knives. We would find them tucked into the cushions of several sofas. When I heard him whisper "It wouldn't hurt much," I turned to find him gently poking a knife on his arm without piercing the skin and reported this to his psychiatrist. A few days later, when I found a knife under our mattress, I called his psychiatrist again who instructed me to get Rick immediately to the emergency room.

Once again, off to Fairfax Hospital where we waited for hours. After being escorted to an exam room, I had to corral Rick for an hour to prevent him from escaping out the door. Upon examination, the doctor admitted Rick to the psych ward. I still remember the surreal vision of walking down the corridor of the psych ward and seeing Rick in a room without a bed and only blankets on the floor, which I was told is customary for patients considered as suicide risks.

Twenty-four hours later, they moved him into a room for evaluation. Afterwards, his treating psychiatrist told me he did not know what was wrong with Rick, but they were experimenting with lots of meds, trying to "fire up his neurotransmitters." They kept recommending electroshock treatments (ECT). I resisted.

After a few days, the psychiatrist in the hospital ordered neuropsychological testing. The neuropsychologist assigned to Rick's case had known him professionally and shared that he had been impressed by Rick's once characteristic charisma. Now, he admitted: "Rick is just a shell of that man." His memory center seemed intact, so Rick could recall both short and long-term memories, which perplexed us all until several rounds of neuropsych evaluation pointed to his brain issues.

Eventually it would be revealed through additional expensive and time-intensive neuropsychological testing, that the executive skills/decision-making center of Rick's brain showed deficiencies.

What Is Neuropsychological Testing?

Neuropsychological evaluation is an assessment of how an individual's brain functions, which indirectly yields information about the structural and functional integrity of his/her brain. This series of tests evaluate functioning regarding: intelligence, executive functions (such as planning, abstraction, conceptualization), attention, memory, motivation, mood state and emotion, language, perception, sensorimotor functions, quality of life, and personality styles.

The referring doctor requests the test administrator to specifically evaluate regarding the specific symptoms and complaints and from observations made during the interview and test administration. The scores on these tests are compared to healthy individuals of a similar demographics (e.g., of similar age, education, gender, and or/ethnic background) and to expected levels of functioning. By evaluating all the data from the comprehensive evaluation, the neuropsychologist determines patterns of cognitive strengths and weaknesses, and understands more about the individual's brain functioning to provide a thorough, comprehensive evaluation.[1]

Had those neuropsychological tests been part of his earlier diagnostic testing and interpreted through the lens of a neurotoxic illness, it may have eliminated incorrect assumptions that Rick was suffering from a psychiatric illness. Instead, the examiner's theory was that Rick was dealing with depression brought on by his disabling condition, and his suicidal tendencies were the result of believing the condition might be permanent. Again, another instance of the tale of the blind men and the elephant.

The psychiatric team encouraged electroshock treatments in hopes it might "snap" him out of it. Although I did not think that was the issue, I remained open to possibilities that something might work. At a point of desperation for answers and against my better judgment, I reluctantly agreed to a course of ECT treatments.

After his second ECT, when the technicians wheeled Rick back into his hospital room, I leaned over his bed and heard him whisper, "Nothing is working. Nothing is working."

The Lifesaving Gift of Synchronicity

Later that day, as Rick lay motionless in his hospital bed, barely able to move or speak, I received a phone call from Arnold Sanow, coauthor of our book, *Get Along with Anyone, Anytime, Anywhere.* During the call, Arnold mentioned meeting a woman named Cindi, whom he had recently consulted with about her interest in professional speaking. He explained that she also suffered from a debilitating, chronic illness that sounded strangely familiar to Rick's. Cindi wanted to share the research she had recently come across and I invited her over to discuss her experience.

Cindi arrived with a stack of documents and a book, *Desperation Medicine*, authored by Dr. Ritchie Shoemaker, founder of the Center for Research on Biotoxin-Associated Illnesses in Maryland. Shoemaker's work was exclusively dedicated to those suffering from illnesses resulting from mold, Lyme disease and other biotoxins.

Biotoxin research has revealed that about 25% of the population have a certain genotype that makes them especially vulnerable to autoimmune disorders when triggered by environmental agents. Genetically prone to be poor detoxifiers, they are primed for a condition now recognized as the previously mentioned CIRS. If you have a susceptible genotype, and an abnormal VCS test (described below), you are very likely to show the laboratory abnormalities seen in CIRS. This condition appears to occur only in the genetically predisposed. More details are highlighted in the next chapter.

Within the hour, I asked Cindi if she would come with me to the hospital. Fully understanding the degree of Rick's suffering, she agreed and together we headed to the hospital. Coincidentally, Rick's attending psychiatrist was just making his rounds. Cindi had come prepared with a stack of research on toxin-associated illnesses. The doctor admitted he did not know what was wrong with Rick and he welcomed new information that might prove helpful.

At Cindi's suggestion, he authorized a simple eye test, the Visual Contrast Sensitivity (VCS) administered by computer, a simple screening for neurotoxin exposure. Rick's responses indicated the likelihood for toxic exposure. Now we had more confirmation as to what was at the root of Rick's medical mystery.

Page by page, *Desperation Medicine* perfectly described many of Rick's symptoms. I read the book out loud to Rick and about how mold, Lyme disease, and other biotoxins can lead to depression, anxiety, panic attacks, behavioral changes, and many other symptoms not typically evaluated from an organic perspective.

While reading a paragraph stating that many patients diagnosed with depression, anxiety, multiple sclerosis, and other conditions, may be suffering from biotoxin illness as the root cause, Rick's hospital mate, Tom, pulled back the curtain that separated their beds and declared, "I've been diagnosed with all of them over the last 10 years. I've had regular ECT treatments for years! My house has mold in it."

Wow! Lightbulbs were going off in my brain. This might be why Tom had been dealing with chronic brain issues, too! Dr. Shoemaker referred to biotoxin illness as a "silent epidemic," and estimated that 1 in 4 people are genetically compromised toward developing illnesses related to biotoxic exposure. Because this research was neither embraced nor well-understood by conventional health professionals, I thought about how many patients were being diagnosed incorrectly, receiving tests that did not point to the root causes of their illnesses, and receiving treatments and medications that only treat their symptoms.

Now having more documentation that toxicity may be at the root of Rick's symptoms, I instructed Rick's psychiatrist to stop ECT and begin the detoxification protocol outlined by Dr. Shoemaker, which helps to bind the toxins in the colon and remove them from the body. While Dr. Shoemaker's protocol held promise and a lot more hope, Rick's psychiatric team insisted on more ECT treatments. My intuition sensed that these treatments were not a likely path to healing his condition and they were discontinued.

Rick's psychiatric team was unfamiliar and even suspicious about Shoemaker's research and protocol. For the protocol to be administered, Rick had to be transferred out of the psych ward and supervised under the care of an internist. They also immediately started Rick on medication that the biotoxic research team had found helpful in binding toxins and purging them from the body.

Within a few days, Rick noticeably improved and became more alert and active each day. Upon discharge, the nurse gave me instructions to follow-up with the neurologist who was regarded as an expert in environmental issues and toxicology. Coincidentally, it was another doctor with whom Rick had worked professionally on a client case a few years earlier.

Perfect, I thought! Now, we have a local expert with whom we could consult and who was likely familiar with the groundbreaking research from the Center for Research on Biotoxin-Associated Illnesses (CRBAI), eliminating the need to travel hours away to Maryland's Eastern Shore. As we would later learn, he was not at all familiar with it.

Rick was looking and feeling so much better the day he was discharged—another seeming miraculous turnaround. He was so improved that he was able to attend dinner at my mom's favorite restaurant in celebration of her birthday. I was feeling ecstatic. We toasted to the good health for all.

I thought he had turned the corner and it would be smooth sailing back to health. However, I soon realized that my optimism was short-lived.

Chapter 5
A Toxic Illness

Prescription for Disappointment

February 2005

Rick's treating neurologist, Dr. P., suggested a sleep study, believing that sleep apnea might be one of the causes of Rick's issues. However, I was more eager for Rick to receive the blood tests outlined in Dr. Shoemaker's book, *Mold Warriors*, which I hoped would prove enlightening. Dr. P. reviewed the blood test list and gave us a prescription for all of them. We headed off to the lab for more vials of blood to be drawn. But this time, it would include testing for specific markers of biotoxin exposure.

When the lab results became available, we returned to Dr. P.'s office, anxious for his interpretation. I especially wanted the results for melanocyte-stimulating hormone (MSH), since a low reading was one of the biomarkers associated with biotoxin illness—Chronic Inflammatory Response Syndrome (CIRS).

When Rick's MSH levels came back clearly deficient, Dr. P. did not understand why I was especially concerned about this marker. While we were in his office, Dr P. called Rick's treating psychiatrist at the hospital to say: "His wife is all upset about her husband's low MSH level, which as we both know is important to skin pigmentation." It was becoming clear to me that Dr. P. and Rick's psychiatrist were not familiar with the idea that MSH can be a key player in chronic inflammatory illnesses. I could not understand why; Dr. P. had served as an expert witness on Sick Building Syndrome (SBS) cases, and it seems he should have been familiar with this biomarker.

What's so Important about MSH?

MSH is the "boss" of regulating many of the body's complex different systems. Low MSH is a key indicator of biotoxin illness. The disruption of MSH typically creates a "trio of misery" with patients often left fat, fatigued, and fighting pain.

Dr. Shoemaker explains, "This hormone—probably the most important one that most people haven't heard of—has been unwisely neglected by modern medicine despite being involved in many key functions."[1] MSH is an incredibly active hormone, regulating many functions and controls many of our innate immune responses. In biotoxin patients, when MSH is disrupted, the source of all normal regulation of nerve, hormone and immune function, the cascade of symptoms of biotoxin illness appear.

When MSH levels are low, chronic fatigue follows. Due to cytokine damage, biotoxic patients usually develop leptin resistance, increasing the storage of fatty acids in the fat cells. When you are high in leptin, you store fat and face a steep challenge to lose it.

Dr. Shoemaker notes the connection of MSH to pain: "Low MSH also means low endorphins. Without the 'natural opiates' produced by the brain, the body has no way to shut down responses to pain stimuli ... When MSH is low, chronic pain follows. Exposure to toxins in genetically susceptible patients causes increased cytokine production (inflammation) reducing MSH, resulting in an endorphin deficiency that changes the patient's **perception** of pain."[2]

MSH deficiency also impacts the immune system and the ability of white blood cells to respond to fighting infections. Infectious diseases often last longer with more symptoms.

As noted in CRBAI materials, MSH is to a biotoxic patient as insulin is to a diabetic, yet MSH is no longer available in the US to replace MSH not produced in the body. This means that an estimated 1 in 4 people are genetically compromised and cannot process out mold, toxins from Lyme disease, recluse spider bites, and other biotoxic agents, which cause reactions leading victims down the multi-symptom, multi-system "Biotoxin Pathway." They are frequently diagnosed with depression and/or one or more of the now 100 labels given to autoimmune disorders, such as Chronic Fatigue Syndrome, Sick Building Syndrome, fibromyalgia, and others. This process leads to autoimmunity.

This illness is not revealed through regular diagnostic tools and therefore escapes proper diagnosis. Patients are usually put on a regimen of anti-depressants, anti-anxiety meds, and pills for the headaches, gastric distress, nerve pain, restless legs, and other maladies that coincide with this syndrome. However, these do not address the underlying causes. As the inflammatory processes of the cytokines increase, the afflicted experience intensified symptoms without relief, sometimes even leading to suicide ideation. Patients are in such misery that as time goes by and nothing works—and they feel so sick, chronically fatigued, and hopeless since conventional treatments are not effective—they might think about ending it all.

I knew then that (as inconvenient as that might be) Rick and I would need to schedule an appointment at CRBAI on Maryland's Eastern Shore. More confirmation from Dr. Shoemaker's groundbreaking research would be worth the trip, as well as offer us a much-needed influx of hope.

After completing pages of paperwork to provide a complete medical history, I was able to secure an appointment in six weeks. I was confident that the CRBAI would be the place where we would get answers. Dr. Shoemaker was its director and ardent researcher who had treated hundreds of patients with toxin-associated illnesses. Since his protocol was getting results, it offered us hope. Hope we desperately needed, since Rick's condition was growing unbearable amid intense physical pain. His care demands were outstripping the capabilities of his group home, meaning I had to tell the care consultant to explore other options.

Respite Rx

March

Operating in a perpetual state of the unknown and dealing daily in crisis-mode, one day I vented to the care consultant about how much my life had changed and how unhappy I was with this new reality. Drained by the toll of all the twists and turns of our life, I blurted out, "I really don't like my life right now!" She responded with something that shocked me: "Sandy, this IS your life. You are responsible for how you respond to everything in it. Now, how are you going to create it?" That was a much-needed slap back to reality—I indeed needed to take responsibility for choosing my attitude during this unexpected detour.

As a professional speaker, I had long emphasized the role of personal responsibility in making choices for our greater happiness and harmony. It was clear that I had to remember to "walk my talk." It was up to me to shift my focus to create moments of joy for my sagging spirit, despite the overwhelming circumstances.

After a year of tumultuous living, it was clear I needed a break—a getaway to lift my spirits and regenerate my energy and optimism. So, I booked a much-needed respite to Costa Rica with my youngest daughter, Stacy, and fun-loving brother, A.K.

At the recommendation of the care consultant, I planned for Rick to spend a few weeks in a small group home in Annandale, Virginia, just west of Washington, DC. We visited the home so Rick could see it in advance of his stay. Surprisingly, he did not resist the idea. I wondered why.

Costa Rica revived my energy as I bathed in the natural beauty of the tropics. I submerged myself one glorious day in hot springs bubbling up from the Mount Arenal volcano, zip-lined across the rain forest canopy, and the next day floated blissfully down a river before soaking in the sun on a white, sandy beach. A few nights at The Peace Lodge overlooking a rain forest canopy, complete with a butterfly garden where I saw the rare, Blue Morpho butterfly species, gave my spirit a lift. Yet, evening phone calls to Rick, in which he described his unrelenting pain, quickly brought me back to reality.

April

Neurotoxic exposures "routinely destroy health, degrade function at home and work, and split once-tender marriages. Some of these exposures eventually can kill, but only after a protracted illness brings a merciful end to long-term suffering from an undiagnosed cause.[3]

Ritchie Shoemaker, MD

Finally, April 5 arrived bringing with it the prospect of hope. It was an anxiously anticipated day involving a four-hour trek to Dr. Shoemaker's office in Pocomoke, Maryland. Because of Rick's frequent state of agitation, I feared a repeat of the episode of his uncontrollable behavior under similar circumstances the previous year. To avoid that possibility, when I arrived at Rick's group home, I gave him a sufficient dose of anxiety-relieving drugs before we hit the road for Maryland.

During the drive, I repeatedly played the CD our friend, a professional singer with the voice of an angel, had made just for us. We listened to repeating tracks of "The Prayer" and "I Believe I Can Fly!" The songs lifted our spirits as we traveled without incident to the Eastern Shore.

Because Dr. Shoemaker had read Rick's detailed history in advance of our appointment, he listed several concerns that would likely be revealed through Rick's upcoming testing and bloodwork. He nailed it! Rick once again failed the VCS test—a reliable screening for chronic inflammatory issues—just as he had the earlier VCS test in the hospital. Rick's complete bloodwork of specific markers confirmed that he had a "dreaded genotype," HLA 4-3-53. It's estimated that only 2-3% of the population have this specific genotype, which makes them highly susceptible to prolonged or recurrent exposure to biotoxins and are more challenged in their recovery process.

Dr. Shoemaker never mentioned this to us at the time, but I would learn years later (while reading his 2010 book, *Surviving Mold*) that this is one of the genotypes that did not show the expected improvements in MSH with any kind of treatment. As he states: "There was just something awful about those

HLA haplotypes; I called them 'the dreaded,' as I dreaded seeing them."[4] Fortunately, for today's patients with more compromised genetics, continuing research has revealed more available treatment options for improved recovery.

Biotoxin exposure in the HLA-susceptible results in imbalanced responses in the immune system and compromises the ability to properly process out toxins. Exposure fires up CIRS, the multi-symptom, multi-system illness caused by neurotoxins.

I'm including both the description of the Biotoxin Pathway and the illustrated chart from Dr. Shoemaker's site, www.SurvivingMold.com offering valuable insights.

The Biotoxin Pathway

Reprinted with permission.[5]

Stage 1: Biotoxin Effects

It all starts when a person is exposed to a biotoxin. In most people, the biotoxin is 'tagged' and identified by the body's immune system and is broken down and removed from the blood by the liver. However, some individuals do not have the immune response genes (HLA-DR genes) that are required to eventually form an antibody to a given foreign antigen. In these cases, the biotoxins are not 'tagged' and remain in the body indefinitely, free to circulate and wreak havoc.

Once present in the body, the biotoxins begin to set off a complex cascade of biochemical events. The biotoxin binds to surface receptors (Toll receptors and many more) in nearly every kind of cell in the body. This recognition and binding of the biotoxin causes a continual upregulation of multiple inflammatory pathways, including production of cytokines, split product of complement, and TGF Beta-1. Biotoxins also directly affect nerve cell function, which is one of the reasons that the symptoms and visual contrast sensitivity (VCS) test are so useful in diagnosis.

Stage 2: Cytokine Effects

Cytokines in turn bind to their receptors, causing release of MMP9 in blood. In the brain, cytokines bind to the leptin receptor, preventing its normal function in the hypothalamus. The blocked leptin receptor will no longer create the initiation of steps that lead to production of alpha melanocyte stimulating hormone (MSH). Elevated cytokines can produce many different symptoms including: headache, muscle ache, unstable temperature and difficulty concentrating. This problem is the disastrous effect of MSH deficiency.

High levels of cytokines can also result in increased levels of important compounds such as I-1 and clotting factors as shown by a von Willebrand's profile. Of importance in cardiovascular health, MMP-9 delivers inflammatory elements from the blood into sensitive tissues and can combine with PAI-1 to increase clot formation and arterial blockage.

Stage 3: Reduced VEGF

The elevated cytokine levels in the capillaries attract white blood cells, leading to restricted blood flow and lower oxygen levels in the tissues (we call this capillary hypoperfusion). Reduced VEGF leads to fatigue, muscle cramps and shortness of breath.

Stage 4: Immune System Effects

Patients with certain HLA genotypes (immunity related genes) may develop inappropriate immune responses which may include antibodies to: gliadin (gluten sensitivity), actin, anca (think ulcerative colitis), cardiolipins (affects blood clotting), and more. Most devastatingly of all, the complement system becomes chronically activated resulting in high levels of C4a.

Stage 5: Low MSH

Reduced MSH production results in yet another set of problems and symptoms. The production of melatonin is reduced which results in sleep problems. Endorphin production is suppressed which leads to chronic and sometimes unusual pain. Lack of MSH can cause malabsorption or 'leaky gut' which further weakens and deregulates the immune system. White blood cells eventually lose regulation of cytokine response so that opportunistic infections may occur or recovery from infections is slower.

Stage 6: Antibiotic Resistant Staph Bacteria

Reduced MSH also allows resistant staph (MARCoNS) to survive in biofilm on the mucous membranes. These bacteria further compound MSH deficiency and the problem by producing exotoxins A and B that cleave MSH, further decreasing the MSH levels. At this point, the downward spiral starts to perpetuate itself.

Stage 6: Pituitary Hormone Effects

Reduced MSH can decrease pituitary production of antidiuretic hormone (ADH) which can lead to thirst, frequent urination, neurally-mediated hypotension (NMH), low blood volume, and electric shocks from static electricity. While sex hormone production is often down-regulated the pituitary may upregulate the production of cortisol and ACTH in the early stages of illness, then drop to abnormally low, or low-normal ranges later.

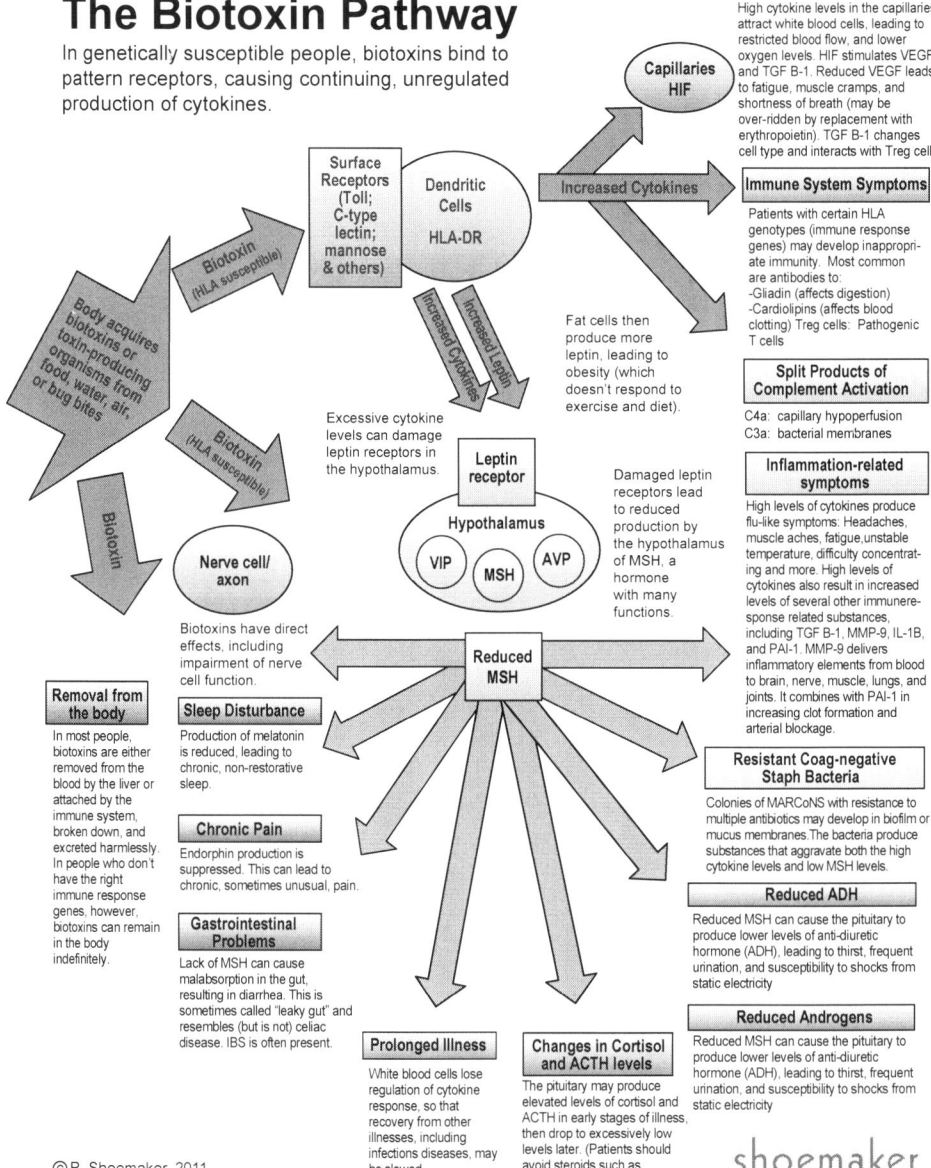

The Biotoxin Pathway

In genetically susceptible people, biotoxins bind to pattern receptors, causing continuing, unregulated production of cytokines.

High cytokine levels in the capillaries attract white blood cells, leading to restricted blood flow, and lower oxygen levels. HIF stimulates VEGF and TGF B-1. Reduced VEGF leads to fatigue, muscle cramps, and shortness of breath (may be over-ridden by replacement with erythropoietin). TGF B-1 changes cell type and interacts with Treg cells.

Capillaries HIF

Surface Receptors (Toll; C-type lectin; mannose & others)

Dendritic Cells HLA-DR

Increased Cytokines

Biotoxin (HLA susceptible)

Body acquires biotoxins or toxin-producing organisms from food, water, air, or bug bites

Biotoxin (HLA susceptible)

Biotoxin

Immune System Symptoms

Patients with certain HLA genotypes (immune response genes) may develop inappropriate immunity. Most common are antibodies to:
-Gliadin (affects digestion)
-Cardiolipins (affects blood clotting) Treg cells: Pathogenic T cells

Fat cells then produce more leptin, leading to obesity (which doesn't respond to exercise and diet).

Split Products of Complement Activation

C4a: capillary hypoperfusion
C3a: bacterial membranes

Excessive cytokine levels can damage leptin receptors in the hypothalamus.

Leptin receptor

Hypothalamus

VIP **MSH** **AVP**

Damaged leptin receptors lead to reduced production by the hypothalamus of MSH, a hormone with many functions.

Inflammation-related symptoms

High levels of cytokines produce flu-like symptoms: Headaches, muscle aches, fatigue,unstable temperature, difficulty concentrating and more. High levels of cytokines also result in increased levels of several other immunere-sponse related substances, including TGF B-1, MMP-9, IL-1B, and PAI-1. MMP-9 delivers inflammatory elements from blood to brain, nerve, muscle, lungs, and joints. It combines with PAI-1 in increasing clot formation and arterial blockage.

Nerve cell/ axon

Biotoxins have direct effects, including impairment of nerve cell function.

Reduced MSH

Removal from the body

In most people, biotoxins are either removed from the blood by the liver or attached by the immune system, broken down, and excreted harmlessly. In people who don't have the right immune response genes, however, biotoxins can remain in the body indefinitely.

Sleep Disturbance

Production of melatonin is reduced, leading to chronic, non-restorative sleep.

Chronic Pain

Endorphin production is suppressed. This can lead to chronic, sometimes unusual, pain.

Gastrointestinal Problems

Lack of MSH can cause malabsorption in the gut, resulting in diarrhea. This is sometimes called "leaky gut" and resembles (but is not) celiac disease. IBS is often present.

Resistant Coag-negative Staph Bacteria

Colonies of MARCoNS with resistance to multiple antibiotics may develop in biofilm or mucus membranes.The bacteria produce substances that aggravate both the high cytokine levels and low MSH levels.

Reduced ADH

Reduced MSH can cause the pituitary to produce lower levels of anti-diuretic hormone (ADH), leading to thirst, frequent urination, and susceptibility to shocks from static electricity

Reduced Androgens

Reduced MSH can cause the pituitary to produce lower levels of anti-diuretic hormone (ADH), leading to thirst, frequent urination, and susceptibility to shocks from static electricity

Prolonged Illness

White blood cells lose regulation of cytokine response, so that recovery from other illnesses, including infections diseases, may be slowed.

Changes in Cortisol and ACTH levels

The pituitary may produce elevated levels of cortisol and ACTH in early stages of illness, then drop to excessively low levels later. (Patients should avoid steroids such as prednisone, which can lower levels of ACTH)

© R. Shoemaker, 2011

shoemaker

Also listed on www.SurvivingMold.com are some of the common symptoms Dr. Shoemaker has documented in his patients suffering from exposure to biotoxins:

Chronic Inflammatory Response Syndrome

- Abdominal pain
- Aches
- Appetite Swings
- Blurred vision
- Comprehension of new information
- Confusion
- Cough
- Diarrhea
- Disorientation
- Dizziness (vertigo)
- Excessive thirst
- Fatigue, weakness
- Focus/concentration issues
- Headache
- Increased urination
- Joint pain
- Light sensitivity
- Memory issues
- Metallic taste
- Mood swings
- Morning stiffness
- Muscle cramps
- Numbness /tingling
- Red eyes
- Sinus problems
- Shortness of breath
- Skin sensitivity
- Static shocks
- Sweats (especially night sweats)
- Tearing
- Temperature regulation or dysregulation problems
- Tremors
- Unusual pain
- Word recollection issues

Rick exhibited many of these symptoms and his biomarkers confirmed that toxicity was at the root of his illness. His long-term, chemical exposures from his childhood, his biotoxic exposures from our mold-infested basements, suspected Lyme disease, and his body's inability to detoxify, proved to be a perilous combination.

Rick's genetics and compromised immune system had caused him to become autoimmune so his body resisted healing, which aligned with Dr. Shoemaker's research. A characteristic of chronic inflammation is a shift of symptoms—their presentation, duration, and intensity, as well as a lack of response to seemingly appropriate medication. Well-meaning doctors prescribe medications to ease pain, improve sleep, calm nerves, reduce depression and other symptoms, which may offer some relief, but none of which get to the core of the problem. This lack of knowledge results in misdiagnoses or delayed diagnoses, meaning untold suffering for those with CIRS and possible permanent damage to vital organs.

Many diagnostic tests from CT scans, sonograms, regular blood tests, nerve conductivity tests, MRIs and other exploratory tools often do not reveal any problems, further compounding the frustration and confusion of CIRS patients, and prolonging their suffering. These tests do not and cannot screen for toxin-associated conditions.

Those afflicted with toxin-related illnesses are indeed sick and tired and research reveals why: the blood flow to the body begins to be restricted at the same time oxygen levels decrease, therefore making it impossible for the person to feel energized. In fact, normal activity will often leave them panting and exhausted. It can take them hours and sometimes days or weeks to recover.

Finally, we had answers and a diagnosis that made sense of it all. Now, Rick's history of neurotoxicity and the pieces of his medical mystery were taking shape:

- Although we were not tracking mold back in the early 1980s, we had lived in a house for four years where the basement flooded after heavy rains or when snow melted after a storm. It was a musty mess! Since we only used the basement for storage, we never resolved the issue. So, mold-infested air and the dangers it presented were unknowingly part of our lives.

- As a home-based consultant, Rick's office was in the basement, where he spent his daily working hours for many years. Then, when my mother came to live with us, she lived in the basement while Rick moved his office upstairs. Since Rick's upstairs office faced due west, and our air conditioning system wasn't effective against intense afternoon sun, he purchased a window air conditioner. Later, after Rick tested positive for biotoxins, professional mold testing confirmed the window air conditioner in Rick's upstairs office contained toxic mold, along with many strains found in the basement. This is the same room which later became my mother's bedroom; she also became sickened with CIRS.

- In the summer of 2003, I remember seeing a red rash on his back, indicating a possible tick bite, long before I learned of the dangers of ticks and Lyme disease. Although Rick did not test positive through the unreliable Western Blot or ELISA tests, his blood work at the CRBAI indicated Lyme exposure was a real possibility. (See Appendix B: "The Ticking Time Bomb of Lyme.")

- Rick had long-term exposure to toxic chemicals: solvents of formaldehyde, benzene, naphthalene, and others while growing up adjacent to his family's leather tanning factory. Their turn-of-the century house contained lead pipes and lead paint. Heavy metals testing from Rick's hair samples and 24-hour urine collection samples indicated high levels of lead, cadmium, aluminum, and other toxic metals.

- Like all of us, Rick also had chronic exposure to 21st century environmental pollutants in air, water, food, and consumer products, including his massive consumption of artificial sweeteners. His preferred diet also contained refined sugars and carbohydrates. Rick's diet was never properly evaluated for its content or any food sensitivities.

Rick was prescribed medication to help bind toxins in the colon for elimination from his body. We felt reassured that detoxification would help to lighten Rick's toxic burden, even though his long-term prognosis was unknown.

Dr. Shoemaker's protocol for clearing toxins with specific medications had been well-documented by the time of our visit. My confidence was growing that Rick's health would soon be fully back on track and yet, there were no assurances. His excessively high inflammation markers combined with his rare genotype presented an uphill battle for full recovery. As Dr. Neil Nathan—a passionate advocate for environmentally mediated illnesses—notes: "Toxins often interfere with the ability of these [detoxification] organ systems to function, paradoxically creating a downward spiral—the more toxic a person becomes, the less able these organs are to get rid of toxins."[6]

For those who are genetically compromised in their ability to process out toxins, the body burden becomes extremely hazardous to their health. As Dr. Dan Watts (whose comments were included in the introduction) asks, "While everyone tests positive for toxins, the real question is what burden does it weigh on individual biology?"

The inflammation, caused by Rick's toxic overload manifested with multiple symptoms, is a common course for individuals who are genetically compromised as poor detoxifiers and who often succumb to what is now recognized as CIRS.

Dr. Shoemaker noted that one of Rick's markers, MMP9 (matrix metalloproteinase-9)—an exclusive marker in biotoxin research at the time and indicative of inflammation—was measured at 966 during our first visit. When he later re-tested Rick, his MMP9 level had increased to 1291! A reference range is between 85-332; anything beyond that and people will suffer at least flu-like symptoms; the higher the number, the greater the inflammation and resulting misery. Dr. Shoemaker said Rick's numbers were some of the highest he had seen in all his research at that time. Rick's genetics were not favorable for alleviating his symptoms, or for a full recovery.

This rampant inflammation from CIRS manifests with multiple symptoms and affects multiple systems. He diagnosed Rick with *toxic encephalopathy*—toxic brain inflammation—now recognized as an autoimmune disorder. This diagnosis encompassed all his symptoms and explained his strange behavior and neurological issues.

Brain inflammation can result from the presence of toxic substances that create an inflammatory response destructive to brain tissue.[7] At the onset of Rick's diverse symptoms, toxic encephalopathy was recognized in isolated medical frontiers, but certainly not mainstream medicine. In fact, the article, "Toxic Brain Injury (Encephalopathy)" by John Upledger, a Doctor of Osteopathic Medicine, details how toxins trigger brain inflammation. Although it appeared in a publication just months after Rick's initial manifestation of symptoms,[8] I only discovered it during research for this book.

> *It generally takes longer to recognize the effects of toxic substances on the brain, spinal cord, autonomic nervous system, voluntary peripheral nervous system. The brain seems to be a keen competitor for the title of slowest responder with the most endurance. What we have been calling "senescent changes in brain function due to normal aging processes" may actually be due to slowly advancing brain inflammation. I refer to that as toxic encephalitis or toxic encephalopathy.[9]*
>
> John Upledger, DO, OMM

Coincidentally, Dr. Watts and his wife were both stricken with a barrage of symptoms in 2004, around the same time as Rick, when little information was available regarding the health hazards of biotoxins and the havoc they generate.

A doctor's personal story with mycotoxicosis (mold illness)

My introduction to the study of mycotoxins began, not as a student or as postgraduate course, but as a patient.

Not much had been written in peer reviewed literature about the serious medical problems associated with toxic mold exposure in 2004. The CDC had not yet recognized mycotoxicosis as a disease entity.

My wife, Sherry, and I had begun to experience symptoms of fatigue and immune deficiency, fungal outbreaks (skin, toenail, vagina, crotch), multiple respiratory illnesses and sinusitis. Sherry developed major GI problems. We had also noticed a musty smell from the air conditioner.

In 2005, our house was found to have *Aspergillus and Penicillium* mold growing around the air conditioner system and into the walls. Shortly afterward, we moved out of the house for remediation. Even though the respiratory symptoms diminished, the fatigue persisted. Sherry required surgery for GI issues, and I developed a TCell Lymphoma.

At the time, there were no physicians in our area to connect the mold in our home to the cause of our medical problems. Following my own reading of Dr. Shoemaker's book, *Mold Warriors,* highlighting medical problems associated with mold toxicity, as well as phone consultations with Dr. Croft (a veterinarian working with mold toxicity as a bioterrorist warfare instrument), we were able to run tests which led to the diagnosis of *Trichothecene Mycotoxicosis.*

Had we not found the root cause of my cancer and Sherry's GI problems, we might well be dealing with those issues today or be dead. As it stands, we were able to rid our bodies of the trichothecenes. We are both doing much better than we were 15 years ago. My cancer is in remission and Sherry's GI problems are stable, thanks to functional and integrative medicine.

—Dr. Dan Watts

Chapter 6
Challenges of an Accurate Diagnosis

Given that autoimmune diseases are often rare and may not be easily diagnosed with blood tests, imaging, and other standard tests, clinicians who aren't familiar with these illnesses can find them perplexing. It's not unusual for truly sick patients to be dismissed by medical professionals as lazy or neurotic ... It can take years to diagnose some of these conditions.[1]

Stanley Finger, Autoimmune Association

Chronic inflammation plays a role in every major disease—dementia, autism, ADHD, mood and behavioral disorders, obesity, autoimmune disorders, cancer, and others. As Neil Nathan, MD states in his book, *Toxic*, "The underlying theme for all of these conditions, whether they are triggered by toxins or infectious agents, is inflammation."[2]

During our long journey to an accurate diagnosis, Rick's physicians dismissed his history of long-term, toxic exposure to chemicals and biotoxins, as well as the research and testing that confirmed these connections. I made a point to provide this history at every appointment. Even after his test results revealed recent, extremely high biotoxic exposure from mold and likely Lyme disease as well, treating neurologists and psychiatrists continued to discount that he was suffering from a neurotoxic connection.

When I shared Rick's high inflammation test results along with the compelling research from the Center for Research on Biotoxin-Associated Illnesses with the neurologist with whom Rick had worked together on client cases, he scanned it briefly, put it on his desk and exclaimed, "We've agreed to disagree."

"No, we didn't," I replied. "You've chosen not to be open to the research."

In fairness to this neurologist, the science of biotoxin illness was relatively unknown at that point, yet with such detailed documentation presented to him, I thought it would have more than piqued his interest to explore such possibilities.

With interest for protecting those who have had their lives turned upside down by biotoxins, people must realize that most conventionally trained doctors are still not familiar with mold illnesses. This means many patients travel similar paths as we did—through multiple revolving doors in medical facilities without producing correct answers, only assumptions.

As Dr. Shoemaker relates in *Surviving Mold*: "On average, my new patients have seen just over *10* physicians, trying to find a diagnosis and/or treatment that actually help. Usually, if you are seeing me, it is because the system failed you. I can't tell you how many of those physicians' medical records show what I call *diagnosis by assumption*."[3]

This was certainly true in Rick's case and perfectly reflected in Dr. Shoemaker's description of many similar caseloads: "If the CAT scan, MRI and endoscopy are normal, not to mention the EMG, spinal tap, sleep study and more, there are physicians (#1) who *assume* that their patients have *psychiatric* problems as an explanation for their many symptoms or they're malingerers or worse. The next physician (#2) who sees the patient reads comments in the medical record like, 'diffusely positive review of systems; all studies normal, stress in life,' and immediately understands the implied assumption: *the patient is a wacko.* The assumption continues: not just that the patient isn't truly ill, but physician number #2 introduces new medications and more tests (they are normal too), essentially making additional diagnosis and treatment decisions based on the original but incorrect assumption. This happens every day in American physicians' offices."[4] Bingo! This is indeed a most accurate recount of our personal experience.

The losses are seismic for patients and their families, shaking up lives to their core. When a patient's treatable illness is ignored and suffers loss of health, job, home, spouse or partner, and the freedom to live and interact with loved ones as they previously had—due to providers' lack of due diligence—it's simply unconscionable. This conflicts with a physician's Hippocratic oath: "According to my greatest ability and judgment, I will do no harm or injustice to them." Grave injustices are currently being perpetuated amongst those who are unaware of, or deny the existence of, biotoxic illnesses.

In 1962, a scientist referred to mold mycotoxicosis [mold toxicity] as "the neglected disease." Decades later, research confirmed that: "The manifestations and disorders in humans caused by molds and mycotoxins continues to be overlooked or unnoticed by many physicians. Each year studies continue to be published throughout the world medical and scientific literature elucidating and explaining the pathological processes and biomechanisms by which exposure to molds and mycotoxins cause sickness in humans ... The exact biological and chemical actions through which these mechanisms unfold is not completely understood ... Science and medicine should continue its work in these areas and bring about the much-needed change from 'the neglected disease' to 'the accepted disease.'"[5]

A more recent publication, the *Handbook of Toxicologic Pathology*, states that "[a]lthough mycotoxin-induced diseases have been recognized for many years, even centuries, recognition of specific mycotoxins as causes of disease is a comparatively recent development. As a result, major knowledge gaps remain to be filled through research for many of the known mycotoxins, particularly the potential human health effects of low-level chronic exposure, identification of biomarkers of exposure, and the effects of mycotoxin interactions."[6]

When a condition is not properly diagnosed, medical errors can further compound issues. Frequently, conventionally trained physicians misdiagnose mold mycotoxicosis, treating it as a bacterial infection and prescribing antibiotics. However, the Toxic Mold Foundation states "the bacteria in your body are necessary to fight off fungal infections. This is like trying to put out a fire with a flamethrower."[7]

Mold illnesses strike all ages of the genetically susceptible. As I write this, a 12-year-old neighbor boy has been suffering for months with difficulty in concentrating, experiencing behavioral issues, headache, fatigue, digestive issues, and serious intestinal bleeding, which sent him to the hospital for testing. His father shared with the doctors early on that he had recently suspected mold in his house and tried remediating it himself. After a series of lab tests revealed no clear diagnosis, a doctor performed a colonoscopy, which showed non-cancerous spots on the walls of his colon. It would take a specialist flown halfway across the country to diagnose those spots as mold spores. His conventional practitioners administered steroids, a common treatment for inflammatory issues, but one that is hazardous to those with compromised genetics for detoxifying mold. As I write these words, he remains chronically ill.

Another problem associated with physicians who are unfamiliar with the complications of biotoxin illnesses is prescribing medications that are harmful to biotoxic patients. Dr. Shoemaker and other physicians familiar with these illnesses, warn against prescribing steroids to patients with a genetic susceptibility to biotoxin illness for the complications that can result. My mother's own experience with complications from that medication are noted in "Our Genetic Roulette Wheel" in chapter 15.

> *It is time to improve medical education in the field of chronic inflammatory responses syndromes for those who arrogantly deny the existence of mold illness.[8]*
> Ritchie Shoemaker, MD

A Neurotoxic Diagnosis and Treatment Protocol

Of all the specialists we consulted for more than a year following the onset of Rick's illness, only Dr. Shoemaker was able to confirm that biotoxic exposures were linked to Rick's inflammation. At long last, Rick received the right evaluation to confirm the severity of his neurotoxic condition, along with a proven protocol to help ease his symptoms and recover from such a debilitating illness.

Rick's history of decades-long chemical exposure, coupled with the confirmation of his "dreaded genotype" that compromised his ability to process out toxins, resulted in massive inflammation and autoimmune reactions affecting his body and brain. We finally had a diagnosis, but his prognosis remained unknown, especially with his "dreaded genotype."

Although the protocol for removing toxins with medications appeared to be working at first, Rick's overall condition was not significantly improving, and I was losing hope. In addition, because of his cognitive impairment and complex health issues, doctors advised he receive 24-hour supervision for his own safety.

By late April, Rick's whole-body pain was horrific and the supervising nurse at the group home said they could no longer manage his care, or the special "no-amylose" diet regimen recommended as part of Dr. Shoemaker's protocol. This is a very strict diet designed to reduce inflammation by avoiding starches and sugar contained in certain carbohydrates. (See Appendix C: "The Forbidden Foods on an Amylose-Free Diet.")

Rick was moved into a skilled nursing facility better suited to follow the restrictive diet. However, I was unable to supervise every meal and he complained of the unappetizing menu with its many restrictions—no sugar, grains, gluten-rich breads, pasta, cakes, cookies, bananas, potatoes, sweet potatoes, peanuts, and others. I sympathized.

With my desire to offer Rick comfort while he was suffering such distress and pain, I made allowances. Indeed, what was delivered on his tray appeared so unpalatable! I reasoned that since he was now residing in a nursing home, away from home and feeling so sick, some "comfort food" might offer him some momentary joy.

Back then, I did not realize how that diet was important for his recovery or I would have insisted on his adherence to it. Again, I was responsible for supervising a condition most health professionals did not understand, and without benefit of their guidance, I struggled in my decision-making.

While I continued to be relatively optimistic, I also needed a healthy dose of realism to address Rick's care needs. Shoemaker's protocol had helped Rick, but his long-term lack of MSH production had serious and likely irreversible effects. We did not know how long Rick's MSH levels had been severely depleted and all of its implications. I reached out to his doctors for guidance.

Summer

Through the late spring and summer of 2005, I continued to correspond with Dr. Shoemaker and Rick's internist, Dr. T. I recounted Rick's difficulty in breathing and speaking, severe electrical sensations in his brain, crushing headaches, fluctuating cognition, extreme weakness, nausea, and stabbing abdominal pains. I questioned his long-term prognosis, seeking insights on how best to plan for Rick's long-term care as well as how best to cope with the life-changing impact on our family and financial future.

Unfortunately, no prognosis could be made since a predictable pathway for treating toxic-related illnesses was not well known then, especially with Rick's genetics. We waited for availability to transfer Rick from the skilled nursing center into a desirable assisted living facility near our home.

When that day arrived, I was eager for Rick to be welcomed by the friendly staff, but upon arrival, Rick began talking gibberish. I wondered if this might be due to the inflammation, to brain damage from toxic assault, or the chemical cocktails he was taking in hopes some drug combination would help. Likely, the stress of being moved into yet another new place played a role.

After all, I wondered, how did he really feel entering another new experience? He had lost so much over the past 15 months, including our familiar way of communicating. He no longer shared many feelings with me. And then I wondered again … Did he know? Did he think about things like we used to explore in the past? Or was the emotional pain from it all, too difficult to talk about?

I later discovered a journal Rick had compiled during this time. It was heartbreaking to read, especially this entry: "This condition is excruciatingly painful and there is no mechanic in sight to do repairs. I hear stories of lost persons where there exists a status called 'rescue and recovery.' Often there is a question as to what shape the individual will be when recovery occurs. My status is distressingly not much different from a year ago. This is one of the reasons I have a DNR code on my chart. "

With his care needs addressed, I began to redirect my energies into professional pursuits and handling all the details that were now my sole responsibility. It was overwhelming at best, but if we had not invested in a long-term health-care policy, the blows from the unexpected would have been even more devastating. (See Part 5, "Strategies for Managing Life's Uncertainties.")

Later that summer, Rick's pain became so severe, the assisted living staff recommended palliative hospice care to administer drugs, such as methadone and others, for pain management. Unfortunately, Dr. Shoemaker was too far away for regular visits or to closely monitor his care. Although Rick's internist worked in conjunction with Dr. Shoemaker by phone, I still felt alone in managing Rick's care, especially pain management, since methadone and the other pain medications prescribed to him could not provide needed relief.

At the doctor's recommendation, I agreed to a medication that had proven to be helpful to some patients with high inflammation. It was expensive and not covered by insurance, which is true for many experimental therapies.

Rick's doctors could not offer much guidance, and not knowing the course of his illness made everything more difficult. Dr. P, the neurologist who had knowledge of environmental issues, told us he had exhausted his medical knowledge and could no longer help Rick. His internist, although open to expanding his understanding of Rick's issues, was not able to offer more pain management beyond its current scope.

My emotions were raw from several near-death scenes when the end seemed inevitable. When Rick's pain became unbearable, we prayed for release. When it subsided for a time, I climbed once again aboard the roller coaster of hope for another trip around the track. The facility advised me to make funeral arrangements.

After nearly a year and a half of scrambling everywhere in search of answers and healing, people reassured me that I had done all that I could. Through the exhausting and confusing journey, I realized the situation was indeed out of my hands and would unfold as it was supposed to do. It was a difficult lesson of letting go of control or expectations. With nothing left to *do*, I could only *be* a loving support for Rick. Our friends, chaplains, ministers, and others surrounded us with their love and support, too.

Chapter 7
Transformational Turning Points

We knew now how essential detoxification was to Rick's healing. Looking back at our journey there were several defining moments that created turning points in Rick's condition. Dr. Shoemaker recognized Rick's need to detoxify and provided medication to that end. In addition, our friends, Lowell and Dotti, introduced us to a whole-body herbal cleansing system specially formulated to release toxins and other impurities. We used this cleansing product throughout the rest of Rick's life, except for the times I was not permitted to supervise his care. (See chapter 19 for more information.)

I also asked the nursing team to begin administering the homeopathic medications for detoxing mold, Lyme disease, and heavy metals, as well as treating other symptoms Rick was experiencing. The medications had been prescribed to Rick in the fall of 2004 by a naturopathic doctor but discontinued when Rick entered the hospital in January 2005.

A week after starting both the cleansing regimen, nutritional therapies, and homeopathic medications in addition to Shoemaker's protocol, noticeable changes took place. Much to the surprise of all who cared for him, Rick's pain level decreased. Not only was he was moving better, flickers of personality and animation burst through. We all believed a miracle was in the making and with continued improvement, Rick was discharged from palliative care for intense pain management in September, although he still resided at the assisted living center.

Relapses and Remissions

September-December 2005

Rick was making such strides! Increasingly optimistic regarding his chances of recovery, I considered moving him home permanently from assisted living. But his good days never lasted long enough. Just when Rick seemed to be improving, he took another nosedive in October. His pain intensified and he experienced shortness of breath, wrenching stomach pain, and diarrhea. I put my plans to bring him home the end of the month on hold.

In November, a nurse called to say Rick was having severe breathing issues and chest pains. They rushed him to the hospital by ambulance.

Since I was now well-versed in Dr. Shoemaker's diagram of the Biotoxin Pathway,[1] I remembered that CIRS patients are subject to a reduction of vascular endothelial growth factor (VEGF), which supports the delivery of oxygen. Once at the hospital, Rick's oxygen levels were monitored, and he registered as fully oxygenated. They inserted an oxygen tube into his nose—standard procedure for people complaining of shortness of breath—but getting more oxygen into his lungs was not the issue.

With Rick's low VEGF production, his body's ability to get oxygen delivered to his blood vessels was compromised. I explained this to the nurses and the attending physician, but they repeatedly told me, "We just treat symptoms, not diagnose." I always hoped in all our visits to medical facilities, someone would be receptive to exploring the research I shared with them.

What does VEGF have to do with it?

CIRS unleashes cytokines, those inflammatory agents which knock out the control of production of VEGF, essential for brain development and repair. Inflammation ultimately reduces the flow of blood through the capillaries, which means oxygen delivery is compromised. In healthy people, without the inflammatory action of cytokines, blood vessels are dilated, increasing oxygen flow. Biotoxic illnesses suppress VEGF production, which further adds to the symptoms of fatigue, cognitive impairment, shortness of breath, muscle cramps and aches, and poor recovery from even mild exercise.[2]

On Thanksgiving of 2005, our family enjoyed a feast on hospital trays with all the culinary tastelessness of hospital food. However, we were grateful that Rick still had made progress since the previous Thanksgiving.

We all learned the hard way that a body genetically unable to dispose of toxins can alternate between relapse and then a remission of symptoms. We never knew what the day would bring, so planning activities became contingent upon Rick's health status at that moment.

Finally, they discharged him with instructions to continue using oxygen. He did for a few days, without much effect.

Not this! Not Now!

While dealing with all of Rick's health issues and rounds of continuing appointments, I began noticing fluttering sensations traveling down my face and near my ear. I just thought it was a result of all the stress I had experienced. Yet, the disconcerting sensations persisted and my friend, Allie, who had recently undergone brain surgery, urged me to seek answers.

In between all the appointments for Rick and my mom, I finally consulted with a neurologist and had an MRI. I requested a copy of the radiology report, a habit I fortunately developed during Rick's care. As I scanned the report, my heart dropped.

There is a 12 mm mass encasing the left fifth cranial nerve on the left side of the pons. The mass enhances markedly following the intravenous administration of gadolinium and extends caudally through the level of the IAC. The findings are likely those of fifth nerve neuroma ...

I had a brain tumor.

I called the neurologist (another doctor with whom Rick had worked cases) to clarify the report and he reported: "All is well."

"All is well, doctor? What is this 12 mm mass near my fifth cranial nerve?"

"Oh, yes. We need to monitor that."

Apparently, he had barely given my MRI report a cursory glance. As a neurologist, how did he "miss" seeing a brain tumor in the radiology report? If I had not requested a copy of my lab report, I would not have known there was even an issue, except of course for the continuing flutterings and headaches, which I likely would have attributed to stress.

There is never a good time for news about having a brain tumor, but it was particularly bad timing since I was the primary caregiver for both my husband and my mother. I didn't know if I would need brain surgery. This was another unforeseen circumstance to factor into other mounting concerns, adding to my feelings of being overwhelmed (I write more about the complexities of caregiving later in this book).

As for that brain tumor, doctors have monitored it annually. By 2015, I had undergone 28 targeted radiation treatments to stop its growth. An MRI in 2020 revealed it was stable and I remain hopeful that it will be permanently reduced, or even better, miraculously disappear.

January-May 2006

Rick's condition had worsened again, and he experienced more shortness of breath and increased body tremors, as well as unbearable pain. By February, he was showing some improvement, but he continued to experience up-and-down days with fluctuating symptoms.

Living in the moment had become our way of life. Since he looked remarkably well, on the day of our church's "Spring Fling," I asked Rick if he would be able to attend. Rick and I had not danced together since that Strauss waltz a few years earlier in Vienna, Austria, when our lives had a totally different rhythm. With his ever-changing symptoms, he wasn't sure until 5:00 p.m. the day of the event if he could make it. But we did!

Surrounded by the many loving friends whose spirits continually sustained us, Rick and I soon found ourselves once again gliding across the dance floor. This time, the music was a song Rick and I had listened to repeatedly during those very dark days, "I Believe I Can Fly!"

Buoyed by the belief that Rick was getting better, I arranged to bring him home.

Homecoming

June

After 15 months residing in several facilities, we moved Rick back home on June 15. He said goodbye to the staff and his friends at The Gardens as I gathered up his belongings. We were off to begin a new chapter through uncharted waters. A few days later, we stood on the stage at our church, offering our gratitude for all the support we had received from our congregation and thanking everyone for their prayers and assistance. There were tears as everyone rejoiced in Rick's seemingly miraculous recovery.

This would be a new dance for us, but I was determined we would find a way to come to terms with it all. I encouraged Rick to find ways to be of service. With both Stephanie and Stacy home for the summer, we all took strides to adapt to a new cadence. I hadn't been with Rick 24/7 for more than a year and hadn't observed him 'round the clock, nor had I received any feedback from doctors to make me question my desire to move him back home. Doctors did not give me any insights as to what to expect or to be aware of since they weren't certain of his affliction. I naively believed he had returned to the land of the living with a desire to jump back into life.

Admittedly, it felt strange to have him back home, looking and sounding like the husband and father we all had missed for nearly two years. Rick felt a strong desire to be productive and resumed the task of paying bills, as he had done so expertly in the past. I was especially eager to take that responsibility off my plate, and I erroneously believed his brain was now working as it had before.

In filtering through his office files, Rick came across a folder filled with testimonial letters from attorneys, thanking him for the expertise he had provided on their cases. Letter after letter stated how his research and testimony was a major factor in winning sizable awards for their clients. That must have served as the motivating factor to get back to work and be productive by re-opening his vocational rehabilitation consulting business. He started making calls and sending emails to colleagues. His desire to return to his field became compelling. He even renewed his driver's license.

As the coauthor of *Get Along with Anyone*, my intention had always been to "walk my talk" in our marriage, including showing my full support. At this point, I supported his desire to reconnect with colleagues and find some way to be productive.

Rick also attended conferences in Phoenix, Williamsburg, and Philadelphia. I wanted him to pursue whatever would bring him the fulfillment he deserved after such a tragic detour. He appeared to be back on track, but I was not at those conferences to observe how things went. Later, I discovered there was plenty of reason for concern.

Chapter 8
The Unraveling of a Beloved Man

On the Loose ... Without a Safety Net

July-August 2006

With wonderful memories of our vacations together, Rick suggested a getaway to Asheville, North Carolina. After all, during much of the last two years his world outside our home had been limited to hospitals, nursing homes, and assisted living facilities. Prior to Rick's illness, he enjoyed planning trips, so I encouraged him in this role. In July, Rick and I set out on our road trip to western North Carolina, singing the lyrics to familiar oldies as we traveled. Yes, this was how I remembered us! For a brief slice of time, it seemed like the good ol' days were back.

Asheville surprised us with its vibrant, quaint downtown. We found ourselves at a nostalgic Woolworth's lunch counter, sipping on our ice cream sodas and looking at the real estate bulletins. We were now considering a smaller house with less maintenance and no stairs to climb, since Rick still had some movement issues. Both of us really liked the Asheville vibe and thought it might be a charming place to move.

During our visit to the majestic Biltmore estate, we joined a group in the cellar at the winery. While the guide was giving us details about wine pairing, Rick struck up a loud conversation with a woman next to us, an annoying distraction for everyone now straining to hear the guide. When he dropped his wine glass and it shattered into smithereens, I was embarrassed by his loud and obnoxious behavior, which was so unlike the courteous gentleman I had known for so long.

Later that evening, he fell unconscious next to the toilet in our hotel room. Fortunately, I was able to get him up and into bed. The next morning, he wanted to go downstairs to have his complimentary breakfast before I was ready, so I told him to go ahead. When Rick returned, I noticed he was barefoot and had forgotten to put on his shoes. My optimism instantly dissipated. I realized Rick was still dealing with major neurological issues.

When we returned home, I came across a large, plastic bag stuffed with unpaid, overdue bills Rick had secretly hidden. I could no longer overlook or dismiss my observations, knowing that would be disastrous.

Buoyed by our Asheville getaway, Rick contacted a real estate agent to begin exploring buying a home there. His strange behavior coupled with the bag of unpaid bills jolted me back to reality—there was no way I could feel confident buying property. The more I resisted, the more he insisted, and we got wedged into non-negotiable corners.

Before his illness, Rick and I would always find ways to deal with our differences. Now, we could not find any common ground. Rick warned me if I did not go with him to Asheville, he'd fly there without me. As a last-ditch effort, Lowell, our trusted friend, convinced him to attend couples counseling. If he would not listen to either Lowell or myself, maybe someone else could get through to him.

Even with an excellent facilitator, it's impossible negotiating agreements when one of the partners is neurologically impaired. However, the therapist provided a scenario that we both found acceptable—we would return to Asheville together to view properties, but with the caveat that we would not purchase anything yet. I contacted the real estate agent in advance to inform him of the situation and begged his support, to which he reluctantly agreed.

Unfortunately, the agent showed us several highly desirable properties. Rick wanted to buy one. I also had a private conversation with the lending agent and requested that he alert me if Rick ever contacted him. I told Rick I had changed my mind about wanting to move, but I was fearful that he might try negotiating a contract without my knowledge. A few months later, after Rick withdrew my power of attorney and I had no legal means to stop him, that fear became a reality.

Blackouts with a License to Drive

During that summer, Rick's therapist told me that Rick had been in an unreported auto accident. His car was damaged on both sides, but he lied about it, saying someone had hit him. I became increasingly concerned with his driving. Soon after, when Rick passed out behind the wheel in the parking lot at a mall, an employee called the rescue squad. When I arrived, the EMT said, "Keep this man off the road!" Rick just brushed aside my concerns, saying, "I won't hurt anyone."

Rick continued to drive against my wishes, and I begged each of his doctors to provide me with a document stating that Rick was unable to safely drive. All they offered were admonitions. Rick promised each one he would not drive, but since he did not want to be chauffeured, he never kept his promises.

Since doctors' warnings were not stopping him, I had to report him to the department of motor vehicles, fully aware that taking legal action would have profound repercussions on our marriage. Rick screamed, "Go ahead! Call the DMV!" I did, which further fueled his rage and animosity. I was shocked to learn that it was not an immediate revocation. There was a process, involving more paperwork, which took months to finalize. While I waited, I took away his license and hid his keys.

With Dogged Determination

Rick was hellbent on returning to his earlier profession as a vocational rehabilitation consultant. He knew the ability to reason, concentrate, solve problems, and remember various facts were vital in his chosen profession, so he requested follow-up neuropsych testing. Rick contacted the same neuropsychologist who had conducted his earlier tests and with whom he had worked professionally prior to his illness.

This new round of tests once again indicated executive functioning deficiencies, confirming the same area of deficits from his earlier brain SPECT scan. According to the article, "Toxins and Infections" featured on the Neuro-Luminance.com website:

> "SPECT scans of adults labeled as personality disordered often show temporal lobe dysfunction, frontal lobe trauma, or brain toxicity ... Toxins act on the very nature of our personality—turning off motivation, dimming our cognition, and setting off inappropriate impulsivity."[1]

That certainly described some of Rick's uncharacteristic behaviors and personality changes, yet his report only indicated irregularities, not linking toxic connections. However, SPECT scan evidence suggests that a large portion of toxic substance damage has the potential to be reversed; however, the brain does not fully recover. In contrast, lead, carbon monoxide, pesticides, and solvents can cause permanent, irreversible damage to the brain.[2]

I reported Rick's periodic "blackouts" to his neuropsychologist. The neuropsychologist adamantly told Rick not to return to work for at least a year. Following Rick's second comprehensive round of neuropsych testing, the report confirmed:

> "Mr. Strauss' condition renders him fully disabled as far as work return is concerned. Whether he might be able to perform some limited employment function at some distant future time is uncertain. Paradoxically, if that degree of functional recovery is possible, it would only depend upon his ability to emotionally reconcile the certain fact that he is fully impaired at present, may not be "better" later, may be worse if he overstretches his resources trying to fight, or declare his impairment as irrelevant."

Rick was insistent on settling his disability case so he could return to doing what he enjoyed. Witnessing his regular blackouts, impulsivity, and increasingly reactive, irrational communication style, coupled with confirmation from his testing, I fully resisted. Tensions mounted between us.

None of Rick's circle of trusted friends and colleagues could deter him. His behavior became extremely combative, and he developed the mantra: "Don't believe me? Watch me!" He spent thousands of dollars printing up business cards, stationery, securing a website domain, reconnecting with colleagues, and exhibiting at legal conference expos.

September-December

In the fall, Rick wanted another neuropsychologist, Dr. W., whom he had known both professionally and personally for 16 years, to review his second battery of neuropsych test findings. Dr. W. noted the extreme changes in Rick's behavior and told him directly that the test findings were consistent with frontal lobe damage.

The doctor also asked our two daughters and me to respond to the Achenbach scale, a testing device measuring differences in perception of behaviors. From that it was apparent that Rick did not see his behavior as we all did.

Rick became very argumentative with Dr. W. and after a few sessions decided to stop seeing him. I trusted Dr. W. and retained his counsel to air my concerns about Rick's increasingly troublesome behavior. He advised me to keep a log and document everything which would be especially important for gaining guardianship if that became an option. That log later proved to be invaluable.

Brain-Mapping Confirms Deficits

Rick enlisted the support of his long-time, trusted tennis buddy, Dr. D., a neighbor and a psychologist. Two years before taking on the role of Rick's psychologist, Dr. D. had been at Rick's bedside during an especially scary time, when it looked like Rick might be dying. Rick's sessions with him were private but he shared with me that Rick was undergoing neurofeedback brain training and the doctor believed this would work to fully fire up Rick's brain.

In November, Dr. D. performed a Quantitative Electroencephalograph (QEEG)[3] mapping of Rick's brain. Dr. D. stopped by our home one evening to share Rick's results. It indicated Rick had brain deficits in the same area as indicated in his earlier SPECT scan, which also confirmed the results from two complete batteries of neuropsych testing. During our meeting, both Dr. D. and I noted Rick was blacking out, so we cut our meeting short. Right after Dr. D. left, Rick could barely move and needed my help getting to bed.

Rick blacked out again when putting on his pajamas and I observed yet another unusual phenomenon. While standing upright talking to me, he stopped mid-sentence, then bent all the way over with his arms dangling to the floor. He stayed in that position for a minute or two, and then slowly rose, returning upright, without any awareness of having done it. Even stranger, he continued the conversation that had stopped entirely while he was in motion. I stood in disbelief, recognizing that his inexplicable neurological issues were escalating.

A Dizzying Array of Continuing Symptoms

As soon as the neurologist's office opened, I secured an appointment to evaluate Rick's new symptoms of strange movement and extreme dizziness. This was the same neurologist who had assessed Rick after his blackout in the mall parking lot earlier that summer.

The morning of his appointment, Rick was still extremely dizzy, weaving from wall to wall, but I managed to get him dressed, into the car and inside the medical building. Vertigo is one of the many symptoms often accompanying neurological chronic inflammation.

The neurologist conducted a routine exam, as well as a Doppler scan of Rick's arteries, and found nothing significant. But I knew Rick was not well—physically, mentally, neurologically, or emotionally. Each time a new symptom appeared, it prompted renewed fears.

I harbored an unrealistic expectation that perhaps during this exam or maybe the next, there would be a defining, "Eureka!" moment in which the doctor put all the symptoms together and would know exactly what tests and therapies were needed. However, Rick's illness would never be recognized by mainstream medicine until the 11th year of his illness, when he would finally be diagnosed by a neurologist with Lewy body dementia.

While researching additional material for this book, I came across a 2006 article, "The frontal/subcortical dementias: common dementing illnesses associated with prominent and disturbing behavioral changes," by Jonathan T. Stewart, MD, in *Geriatrics*, a magazine for healthcare professionals. I wish this magazine had circulated to more psychiatrists and neurologists' offices when I was seeking answers to Rick' strange behavior and symptoms. It would also have been useful to share with his treating psychiatric team who suspected Rick was afflicted solely with a bipolar disorder. The article adds further credibility to Dr. D.'s evaluation of Rick's QEEG test, demonstrating "relative slowing in the parietal and occipital EEG and neuropsychological testing confirmed frontal and subcortical deficits."

The *Geriatrics* article provided such insights:

"More remarkably, recent memory may be only mildly impaired or even completely normal, often making it difficult for the family or physician to appreciate that the behavioral changes are indeed related to a dementia ... Often, behavioral changes (usually loss of drive or disinhibition) are the most prominent feature, leading to incorrect attribution to a functional psychiatric illness ...

"Previously active and energetic patients may give up their usual activities and hobbies, and personal hygiene may suffer. Ultimately, they may spend the entire day watching television or lying in bed and may become quite resistant to any suggested activity; resistiveness to personal care may eventually become problematic ...

"**Damage to the orbitofrontal system:** generally results in the most disturbing behavioral changes. These patients are disinhibited, typically losing their manners and becoming crude and tactless. Flirtatiousness and undue familiarity with strangers is common, as is general impulsivity. As the syndrome progresses, more problematic behavior ensue; petty crimes such as shoplifting may occur and the patient may become combative with trivial annoyances ... These patients are often misdiagnosed as having functional psychiatric illness (often mania or a personality disorder,) a longitudinal history will clarify the diagnosis."[4]

Increasing Concerns for the Future

January 2007

A new year ushered in a never-before-seen personality, one I identified as "Wicked Rick," a complete antithesis to his former self. He was filled with vengeance and disdain, eventually fracturing almost every friendship, family connection, and professional contact. While I believed it was all related to his brain issues, that did not lessen the distress his behavior created among friends, family, and professional associates.

My confidence in finding new ways to manage our relationship faded as tensions between us escalated. The fact that I had filed paperwork to have his driver's license revoked was a constant source of his resentment. During the first week of January, Rick found his keys and drove away. I called the police and asked that they be on the lookout for him, thinking they would take immediate action. However, the paperwork for revoking a driver's license takes months to process, so there was little the police could do.

Days later, while on our way to church, Rick exclaimed, "I want to report the insurance agent who took me off our auto policy!"

"Can you please just let it go?" I asked.

Rick responded by angrily shouting, "Stop the car!"

After jumping out at the stoplight, he refused to get back in. Since we were a few blocks from church, I drove on, thinking Rick would soon arrive. He never showed up, instead calling a taxi to take him to a nearby mall.

After this incident, Rick continued to withdraw from my daughters and me, mostly staying in the basement on his computer or watching TV. To be honest, we were relieved to have some physical and emotional distance from his abusive behavior.

It was clear that our family desperately needed some time apart. Traveling had always been a way for us to bond and with Rick's illness creating such stressful living conditions, a trip would provide us with a much-needed escape. With that in mind, I planned a two-week getaway to New Zealand with our daughters and my brother, A.K.

Fortunately, our long-term insurance policy would provide for Rick's care while we were away. We made plans at the assisted living facility, conveniently located directly across the street from our church, so our friends and ministers could visit him. These connections would be especially valuable while I had some time away to sort things out.

Stripped of All Legal Rights

January 30

A week before we were scheduled to leave, Rick and I walked into Sunrise Assisted Living for me to sign papers and provide the deposit. Instead, Rick asked for a private meeting with the admissions director while I waited for more than an hour. What was going on? To my surprise, Rick had his own plans in mind. He told them he had revoked my power of attorney (POA) and was now in charge of his own care. The plans that I had carefully put in place so everything would go smoothly while we were away collapsed in an instant.

My steps to revoke his driver's license had been a devastating blow to Rick's desired independence. He believed that he could return to work. Since I could not support that decision, and unbeknownst to me, he had revoked my POA so he could make decisions for himself. To achieve this, Rick had to pass a mini-mental test. Ironically, he persuaded his internist of two years, Dr. T. (who was aware of Rick's medical history), to perform the test. As he had often in the past, he had no trouble passing the latest one. His brain issues were not about short-term and long-term memory—the focus of the mini test—but related to his behavior, executive functioning, and decision-making skills. While all were severely compromised, this test did not evaluate them.

After learning from the admissions director what Rick had done, I called Dr. T. to vehemently protest. He responded that while he was fully aware of Rick's debilitated condition, he had passed the competency test needed for documentation. That is all Rick needed to revoke my POA.

That evening, Rick called a family meeting and invited our friend, Brenda, to attend. He did not know that we had already been informed of the action he had taken. Pacing the floor, Rick announced that he was moving out that night "never to return! He would only reveal that he was moving to "an undisclosed location."

While Rick packed up that evening, Stephanie and I grabbed credit cards and copied passwords, which enabled us to later track his whereabouts and contacts with others. He left the next morning around 7:00 a.m. by taxi. Fortunately, Rick had shared his location with our church ministers; however, ministerial confidence meant they could not ethically reveal his location to me.

Now, Rick was on his own, with no one supervising his care or safety. Fortunately, our church members and friends recognized the gravity of the situation and provided a supportive network. Before leaving for New Zealand, I proceeded to outline pertinent details of Rick's illness as background for them:

> "Due to his compromised impulse control, I have no assurances of his behavior at any time and simply reel in the reality. I have observed a continuing string of bizarre behaviors and have stood by him through them all. I was instructed by experts dealing with this type of brain injury to take action regarding his driving, as well as having to handle other matters.
>
> Although the tests used to determine competency are insufficient for his specific brain issues, he is considered mentally competent according to Virginia law, which puts others and himself at risk. You have all been extremely supportive and appreciate receiving any information related to his condition since I am no longer able to supervise his care.
>
> Rick is in denial of his condition and moving forward with plans since he believes he can rise above his disability. Everything I have received from experts confirm his condition is irreversible. Yet, because his judgment is clouded, and I am now unable to protect either him or our resources, I ask for your help since I've been stripped of legal protection.
>
> This puts our family in jeopardy, and I sincerely appreciate your help in keeping me updated, for my ears and eyes are no longer able to supervise Rick's actions."

The night before the girls and I left, Rick revealed he was staying at a nearby motel. I had a surreal visit with him, recognizing that the man I had once known was gone and the beautiful history we shared was now a mere memory. Rick explained that he had plans in place for his care for the two weeks I would be away, but he refused to share them with me. Fortunately, the church ministers knew where he was and the precarious nature of his situation.

A Relentless Reign of Worry and Fear

February

As the girls and I were boarding the plane for New Zealand, Rick finally took my call. Somehow, he had gotten himself to Sunrise, where I had tried to arrange for him to stay. He didn't understand why they weren't expecting him! Of course not—he had cancelled all those well-laid plans! Fortunately, they had a room available, and I left, somewhat relieved Rick would be safe while we were out of the country for two weeks.

However, I was not able to truly relax on the trip—the whole point of our getaway. Every time I checked emails and phone messages, there was something unexpected that had to be dealt with immediately. Since I had cancelled all joint credit cards, I was alerted that many personal and business-related expenses could not be processed.

When we returned home two weeks later, Stephanie and I noticed Rick's car was gone. Rick left us a note, indicating that his car had been towed to his new home in an apartment complex a few miles away. However, neighbors told us that Rick had driven off in his car. Since the car was registered solely in his name for his business, I could neither legally touch it, nor install a GPS to track him. Rick was now driving an uninsured car without a license.

One of our good friends from church had helped Rick move his things from the house into an apartment—a very strategic move on Rick's part, since he didn't want me supervising his activities. Although I had had the foresight to change the locks on the house when Rick moved out, he had somehow figured a way to gain entry while I was away. Now on top of everything else, I felt unsafe in my own home.

Rick invited Stephanie and me to his apartment the day we returned from our holiday. I was angry and even more afraid of what this new reality meant. An attorney advised me to initiate divorce proceedings, since Rick's aberrant behavior and illegal driving could put me in legal and financial jeopardy, should he have an accident.

Although I had cancelled our joint credit cards the day Rick moved out, he had credit cards in his own name. And, without a POA, I had no access to his accounts. It would not be long until I realized just how irresponsible he had become financially.

Since he was now living alone, Rick's formerly healthy diet, previously supervised by me or the residential facilities where he lived, was a thing of the past. He stocked his kitchen with diet drinks, processed foods, three large boxes of artificial sweeteners, popcorn, candy, and snacks.

Rick had gained weight and mistakenly thought substituting artificial sweeteners would help shed some pounds, especially given his raging sweet tooth. However, someone with Rick's genetics for poor detoxification should not be adding to their toxic load by consuming those things.

For a while, Rick allowed me to visit him in his apartment where chaos reigned. Paperwork and clothes were heaped in piles covering the floors. The kitchen floor was spattered with food and scattered with business cards, artificial sweetener packets, and credit cards. During each visit, I'd check to see if his car had been moved. He fiercely denied driving, yet every time the car was sitting in a different parking space. I also witnessed several narcoleptic episodes again where Rick would drift off the middle of a conversation, with no memory of having done so. This was a frightening reality to contemplate—Rick had narcolepsy, was living unsupervised, and driving on a revoked license!

March

Finally, the medical review board completed Rick's paperwork to officially revoke his driver's license. I was grateful that he had not harmed himself or others during the interim. To ensure Rick would be unable to apply for another driver's license, I sent additional correspondence to the DMV, explaining the medical reasons Rick should never be allowed to drive again.

Because Rick had revoked my POA, an attorney advised me to initiate legal guardianship. Mental health laws are designed to protect the patient, except if they are charged with a criminal offense, so both my attorney and Rick's psychologist had advised me to keep a detailed log of Rick's deteriorating condition. I constructed the log from personal observations and communications from his colleagues, friends, and others concerned about his well-being.

My intention through the course of Rick's ravaging illness was to protect and preserve his dignity, his stellar reputation with colleagues, and our financial resources. However, I could no longer shield either Rick or others from his madness. I had to rely on friends and others in their respective professional capacities for Rick's safety. It was an extensive endurance run of stress, patience, and prayers. I am forever grateful for the guidance and support my friends offered. Every connection served as a lifeline.

A Frightening Health Care Crisis ... HIPAAed Out!

April 2007

With Rick's knowledge of HIPAA's protection of his privacy, he reminded his doctors they were not to have any communication with me. However, my attorney told me that did not prevent me from sending correspondence to them. With continuing reports of Rick's spiraling behavior, I kept his neurologist and internist updated with concerns about his safety, mental instability, impulsivity, irrationality, rudeness, and interrupting behavior reported to me by concerned friends.

He sent me an email that he was no longer communicating by either email or phone. I had no way of knowing if he was safe, with the parameters of a legal system that did not offer much safety or protection for individuals in mental distress. It was painful to see him in need of help and not be able to assist him. Adult Protective Services was only available if a person is in imminent danger to themselves or others. How is that defined? Driving a car with confirmed narcolepsy and impaired judgment? Potentially burning down an apartment? Feeling unbalanced? Evidently not.

My hands were legally tied to do anything in a system designed to protect the privacy of unstable individuals, which puts the safety of the patient and others at risk.

***

I am including an entry from my journal because it may possibly resonate to how a loved one's neurological issues extract such a toll upon a once tender relationship.

April 9

It's the morning of our 30th wedding anniversary. Rick used to commemorate this special day with bouquets, poetry, and sweet sentiments. His surprises always made me feel so adored. Today, I notice feelings of dread arising, in anticipation of more unwelcome surprises springing from his brain, filled with its distortions and misperceptions.

I awaken to another email, his words filled with venom and animosity. He blasted it out to everyone on his contact list, as I see names of our friends, family, colleagues, and a few others I do not recognize. I feel angry he has created such a public forum and I am defenseless to protect my integrity, yet there is a part of me that still wants to protect him.

Even though utterly exhausted, I keep trying to respond to this ever-changing reality, constantly created in this world of madness. I feel both betrayed and embarrassed by his behavior, yet also realize his brain does not know what it's doing anymore, and pretty sure everyone on that list knows it, too.

I miss the life we once had and the love and comfort we both provided to one another, thinking it would last forever. Those days have long disappeared. I do not know what he needs anymore, except help I cannot give him. I am exhausted from this endurance run of responding to the next moment of dread or whatever needs handling.

There is no good "us" anymore. Those precious bonds broken from the ravages of craziness. I call out to the Universe for guidance, for strength, for wisdom. How I long to be loved and to feel safe again!

May

Stephanie and I were now living daily in fear, not even feeling safe at home. Rick stalked me by phone and email, threatening to show up at the house and harm us, or himself. His emails to our family become especially disturbing, with subject lines like: "Good-bye, all. I am dying. See you in the after-later." Another subject line noted, "Beaten and left to die by my family," which contained suicidal thoughts or death ideation referencing "my cold body. What will you say when I'm in my coffin tomorrow? Vicious, slanderous, disgusting, disreputable, despicable, diseased lies regarding the physical body that once existed and now is rotting in the coffin."

Despite friends and family who all shared their concerns, Rick listened to no one. He decimated nearly all relationships, no matter the connection. Though obviously a danger to himself and others, the law protected his rights. All I could do was keep a running log and report him to authorities when the situation seemed to warrant it.

Our travel agent told me about Rick's troubling behavioral changes, letting me know that he had asked her about London itineraries. This news escalated my fears of Rick living unsupervised, with a valid passport and traveling internationally. My mind conjured up frightening possibilities.

He had now gone through three attorneys in seeking a divorce. He also contacted former clients who knew him well and recognized he was not the same man. While I was the primary target of attack from his inability to reconcile my need to protect our financial resources from his incapacitated brain, he also directed his fury at Stephanie, who lived with me during this reign of ugliness.

This is a portion of an email Stephanie sent in hopes her dad would see how distorted his thinking had become and how it was especially weighing heavy upon her own heart. It read in part:

> "You always were a man of honor, but your behavior has become less than honorable. That's so sad, Dad. We always looked up to you as a man of strength, but you're not acting strong now; you're acting like a bully. You're attacking us, but it is you who refuse to see that your brain has stirred up all this. You've lost yourself and you're fighting back at those who love and care about you. We see that and know that as truth.
>
> Do you want to regain our respect? Then stop this madness! Be the love that's inside you, the loving Dad we want back.
>
> What do you want us to remember about you, Dad? Then let that shine. A legacy is being remembered for acts of love. That is your legacy. That is your honor and how you will be remembered. Are you being that love in action? Or have those values been discarded from your heart as well? Think about these things. HONOR. LEGACY. I pray your heart knows the way to go for upholding your dad image and how you want to be remembered."

Having counseled Rick for many months and quite concerned about his well-being, Rick's psychologist and friend, recognized the need for intervention. He contacted the authorities again, who advised me to contact Mobile Crisis, a mental health service. Their counselors shared the usual outcomes: If a person with mental issues refuses treatment, and does not seek it themselves, then sooner or later they will get themselves into trouble and into the judicial system. There was little else we could do but wait for either one to happen. Without anyone able to handle his financial affairs, this further jeopardized our respective financial situations. It was just one of many priorities requiring simultaneous attention.

Heartache on Heartache

Included in this section are a few of the entries from my journal and the suggested log needed for securing guardianship. This was important for illustrating the severity of Rick's decompensation, which intensified during his unsupervised living, without his detoxification and nutritional protocols.

It also demonstrates the potential endangerment to personal and public safety by laws designed for the mentally incompetent's protection. This grants them the freedom to choose whether they seek psychiatric evaluation, unless they commit a crime, whereon they will enter the criminal justice system. Lastly, these demonstrate the unpredictable world created by a patient with an inflamed brain and the roller coaster ride for the patient and loved ones alike.

May 11—I hired a private detective upon learning Rick had driven to Charlottesville on a revoked license to exhibit at a defense attorneys conference. He wants to prove he can still work, but one of his colleagues notified me reporting that attorneys found him to be "pitiful" and "acting like a fool." Said one, "He will never get any business."

A manager from the hotel called me with concerns that attendees, exhibitors, and staff had witnessed Rick's offensive, "Dr. Jekyll/Mr. Hyde" behavior. Since I no longer had any legal authority, I told the hotel manager they should call the police.

May 12—The private detective notified me that Rick had checked out of the hotel and assumed he was heading back home. I alerted the police in each jurisdiction Rick would be driving through, letting them know his mental condition and that his license has been revoked. He was stopped by an officer who called for a tow truck, but did not arrest him, which I was told would have allowed for the possibility of getting him into protective custody.

May 13—Rick leaves me a 10-minute voice message, screaming that Mobile Crisis (MCU) showed up for a visit. They called police because Rick was belligerent. According to MCU, although cordial to officers, as soon as they left Rick became combative again. MCU sends police to my house, since they had witnessed his defiant behavior and feared he could do anything. Two officers arrived and then two more. They listened to Rick's voice message and waited for his arrival. In the meantime, his psychologist persuaded Rick not to act on his threats.

May 14—Since Rick has withdrawn my POA to receive payments for his Social Security benefits, these are being suspended until another payee is secured. I implored his doctor to sign a document stating Rick's inability to handle finances to have his benefits restored (the same doctor who originally signed Rick was of sound mind a few months earlier). Another doctor's signature is also required, so I turned to his treating neurologist. They acknowledged the need to retract their earlier competency claims, offering their signatures affirming his incompetence.

May 30—Rick meets with the senior investigator for an impaired practitioner complaint as a licensed professional counselor, initiated by Rick's colleague. In response, Rick sends threatening emails to his colleague and other peers who sent documents attesting to his impairment.

June 4—Upon learning of the death of an attorney's assistant whom he never had met face-to-face, Rick flew to New Jersey to attend her funeral. The attorney called me, saying Rick's behavior was so disruptive he had him escorted out of the funeral home.

June 5—Rick leaves me a 30-minute voice message at 3:00 a.m., which I did not listen to until the next morning. He was "making his dying declaration" admitting "I know I'm not of sound mind." His message ends stating he has a few minutes left on earth. He begins a countdown: 25, 24. 23 ... The recording stops around 15 because my voicemail reached capacity.

When I listened to the message and tried to reach Rick's cell, he did not answer. Oh my God, what a nightmare! Where exactly was he? Was he alive? Did he really kill himself? Around noon, he left a voice message that the police had taken him to a hospital, but Rick walked out claiming some violation of his ADA rights (Americans with Disabilities Act, which he well understood from his career working with disabled clients).

June 6—Rick called Lowell telling him that he was on his way back to his apartment. I was very relieved that he was safe and back in the area.

June 7—Rick emails me, referencing his rights to access our marital home. With Rick's mental instability and unpredictable behavior, I was advised by both my attorney and the police to get a protective order to keep him away.

June 8—I secured the order, preventing any contact with each other by any means. If either of us did, we would be arrested. Later that evening, I received a phone call from a friend who had encountered Rick at the supermarket, screaming that he had a medical emergency and was going to die and needed to go to the hospital. He asked her to call me. I called the supermarket and the manager got him a taxi.

Rick calls me, yelling that he was coming over. I call the police. Two officers arrive and listen to some of Rick's calls. I show them the petition for the protective order, but it was still at the courthouse and had not been officially served. I receive my own protective order, prohibiting me from any contact with Rick by any means.

June 9—I receive a message from Mobile Crisis that Rick's neighbor called police. Mobile Crisis reports Rick had been agitated and belligerent when police arrived.

June 10—The manager at Rick's apartment complex called me after reading a disturbing email Rick had sent and copied him: "If no answer, call 911 and see you in the afterlife ... I will consider taking my life ..."

That evening I received a call from an unknown number. It's Rick. I remind him we were legally unable to communicate, recording the call. He calls again, leaving a long voice message stating that the protective order "had unleashed the nuclear bomb!"

June 11—One of our mutual friends, a receptionist at a law firm, called to say Rick appeared at the attorney's office, promoting his services. She said Rick was "rambling, irrational and getting upset." He was escorted downstairs and left on foot. The police called me after the law office reported Rick's behavior because of their concern for his welfare.

An hour later, Rick's professional counterpart asked whether I knew if he had been attempting to return to work. I told him about the phone call earlier that day. He was grateful for the information, needed for the impaired practitioner case he had initiated.

June 12—I received a copy of an email, drafted by several of his former colleagues who had worked many cases together with Rick, urging him to get needed help. Despite this serving as valuable evidence of Rick's need for guardianship, I am simultaneously saddened that his once stellar reputation helping disabled clients was now so tarnished.

Rick sends a disturbing, disjointed email and a second violation of the protective order. Rick is arrested for violation of the protective order when he contacted me by phone two days earlier.

The detective calls me later in the evening that Rick was released. I received another call from a police officer around 7:30 p.m. that the library had called the police because Rick was being disruptive. The officer asked me to come get him, but I told him of our protective order and that I would be in violation of it, even if I came under these circumstances. So, I immediately called Lowell, and he and Dotti headed to the library.

Lowell and Dotti talk with the officer and agree to be petitioners to get an involuntary commitment for a psych evaluation. They asked Rick to go voluntarily to a treatment center, but he declined. Rick became agitated and was taken by police back to the Adult Detention Center on a public disruption charge. He was processed into the system. Only later I learned that he had put in emergency calls to Dr. T. earlier that day and went to the ER, but left on his own accord.

Following his arrest and intervention of ADC authorities, he was deemed incompetent to stand trial for his disorderly conduct charge, and was transferred to Western State Hospital, a psychiatric facility. Now that he was in the care of the hospital, the protective order was lifted, and I was able to speak with Rick.

He said during his two-hour ride in shackles to Western State hospital, that he had an epiphany. Through his very confused brain, he finally had come to the realization that I had his best interests at heart and asked me to serve again as his power of attorney. However, my attorney advised me to pursue guardianship, since a POA could be revoked again should he became temporarily lucid. With the very insufficient laws regarding mental competency, I could not risk those repercussions.

Chapter 9
A Space to Breathe and a Time to Grieve

Cleaning Up the Chaos

Rick was now safely in protective custody, confined in a psychiatric hospital through the end of 2007. I felt an enormous wave of relief. I was no longer on duty 24-7, exhausted from responding to one emergency after another while having to sort out an action plan in response. I finally had a reprieve from hypervigilance in documenting every symptom, behavior, mood, and the anxiety this elicited.

I began the process of clearing out Rick's apartment. Since Rick had prevented me from visiting him for several months, once I stepped inside, I was overwhelmed by the absolute filth and disarray. The floor was littered with food, pills, bills, scraps of Post-it notes, assorted documents, photos, and credit cards, all mired to a sticky floor or the stained carpet. There were yellow, pink, and blue artificial sweetener packets scattered everywhere.

I began to filter through all his papers and bills to size up priorities. Fortunately, my friend, the organizational genius Dotti, helped me sort through the chaos and decide what needed to be kept, and what should be discarded.

Feelings of sadness swept over me as I saw his collection of family photos—sometimes ten or more of the same ones he had duplicated and scattered everywhere. Rick had lost his health, joy, livelihood, independence, sense of identity, relationships with most of his friends, and all contact with his colleagues. During the period of his most outrageous behavior, many people avoided contact with Rick altogether. Very few would ever call or visit him again.

I grieved for the losses both of us had suffered over the course of this crazy-making time. Beyond the barrage of physical and emotional assaults, perhaps the greatest toll was the obliteration of the relationship we had carefully and lovingly crafted together and sustained for decades. Now, I would soon become his legal guardian, another reality I had never imagined.

In the Gap before Guardianship

I worked with an attorney to share responsibilities with our mutually trusted friend, Reverend Lowell Smith, to become Rick's legal co-guardians and legally manage his affairs, with me acting as the sole conservator. As such, I was required to secure a bond for our joint assets and submit detailed annual accounting reports to the county government. Every penny spent on Rick's behalf—clothes, entertainment, prescriptions, medical and dental bills, nutritional supplements, insurance, outings, and gifts—had to be included in the accounting. In addition to this detailed paperwork for the remaining nine years until his death, I would pay a hefty annual bond on our joint assets. Although I understood why it was necessary, it seemed an unfair drain on our financial resources and an extra burden on my dwindling time and energy.

Until legal guardianship was finalized, I was unable to directly communicate with Rick's treatment team at the state mental hospital. I was concerned they did not have the benefit of his recent medical history and tests. I anticipated securing guardianship about six weeks later, when I'd be legally able to resume supervision. In the interim, Rick's brother, David, served in that capacity. Although I had kept him regularly updated regarding Rick's health status, David had a more limited understanding of his brother's condition.

Now that Rick was under the care of a psychiatric team, I hoped that all the information and research I had gathered over the course of three years, coupled with all the results from his previous functional testing would finally confirm his real issues. I felt relief and optimism.

Fortunately, Rick was assigned to a psychiatric social worker who had also served as a geriatric social worker. She was a welcome source of support and empathy at a time when my grief was overwhelming. I shared some of Rick's medical history with her to get his treatment team up to speed on his unusual case and hoped they would gain a better understanding of the nature of his brain issues.

From the inception of his illness in 2004 until his hospitalization in June 2007, his physicians had prescribed nearly 30 psychotropic drugs, painkillers, or gastrointestinal medications—a bewildering array that likely exacerbated his issues and contributed to his toxic load. Various specialists prescribed him an assortment of medications, based on their individual assessment of the conditions treated within their specialty. I tried to update them all regarding medication changes with concerns of drug interactions, as well as how the drugs he was taking simultaneously contributed to possible adverse reactions, with symptoms that included cognitive impairment.

She recognized that Rick's case was different, noting deficits that indicated his cognitive issues were associated with dementia. However, Rick's treatment team disagreed, convinced his behavior was instead due to mental illness. Unfortunately, she was soon re-assigned, and I lost that connection when I needed it the most—as a new battlefront ensued with Rick's medical treatment team once I secured guardianship.

Although Rick had been admitted to the state hospital in June 2007, I was unable to supervise his care until mid-August when I gained legal guardianship. His team had been administering a combination of drugs to correct chemical imbalances and that treatment was not resolving his issues, but they tried to assure me they would find the right combination that would work. Although they had a long list of other psychotropic medications that Rick had been administered over 3½ years to no avail, by now I was convinced any combination of their drugs was not the answer.

With an expectation that all the evidence that I provided to them would open their eyes to new science, they would surely recognize the revolutionary nature of it, not only for Rick's case but for others under their care and all to follow. This was a great heartache in having it all discredited because the real causes of his symptoms were not being addressed, prolonging, or preventing his recovery.

Our Heartbreaking Reunion

August

The day I became Rick's legal co-guardian, I drove several hours to visit him at the psychiatric hospital in Staunton, Virginia. Of all places, I could never have imagined Rick would end up there. His slovenly appearance shocked me. He shuffled from his room, severely bent over, and hardly able to whisper. He kept pounding his fist against his head and repeating, "I can't get out of my body! I can't get out of my body!" It was unbearable to see him again in such a diminished state.

The psychiatrist assigned to Rick insisted he was bipolar. He vehemently discredited the toxic metals test revealing Rick's high levels of mercury, aluminum, and lead as well as all the specific blood lab biomarkers indicating organic reasons for his illness. He insisted to repeat the same traditional tests that Rick had undergone several times since the inception of his illness without revealing anything significant—these same tests never would. I implored him to request tests and therapies that demonstrated the organic nature of Rick's issues.

Instead, he proclaimed, "We'll fix him up with the right drugs and we'll send him back to you like new."

Chapter 10
A Difference of Opinions

Dismissed, Discredited and Discouraged

It became apparent that my expectations for Rick's psychiatric team to recognize and embrace the organic nature of his condition were futile. I had been optimistic that, at a psychiatric institution devoted to the full spectrum of brain issues, attending doctors would diligently review his case from a wider perspective.

To offer documented evidence of the neurotoxic nature of Rick's condition, I shared all of Rick's previous evaluations and lab tests showing inflammatory markers, which led to his diagnosis of toxic encephalopathy. In so doing, I believed his psychiatric team would provide the needed therapies for Rick's continuing detoxification and nutritional support so decisive to his care. Upon learning of the hospital's presumed bipolar diagnosis, Rick's psychologist, who had administered an earlier QEEQ report in 2006, submitted his report showing brain damage.

However, the doctors disregarded my pleas for an open-minded evaluation. Rick's treating psychiatrist dismissed them, insisting Rick was undoubtedly suffering from brain chemistry imbalances, which could be corrected with medications. Without the detoxification protocols or the nutritional support that had proven so beneficial in the past, Rick's condition worsened during the six months at this facility.

Lowell had stepped forward to assist me getting the right treatment for Rick. We petitioned the hospital administrator for Rick to be put in the hands of a care team more receptive to our wishes, and Rick was eventually reassigned. Yet, the new team also refused to put Rick on the recommended detoxification and nutritional regimen. Instead, they continued pumping him with trials of different psychotropic drugs, none of which seemed to have any positive impact.

The lead psychiatrist who headed up the team that had examined Rick essentially dismissed my concerns as well as all the earlier tests and evaluations from other doctors.

Since Rick was under the authority of Virginia's correctional system, Lowell and I, as his co-guardians, were still legally restricted for influencing his care. Although we had provided records of all of Rick's previous testing, he was still subjected to repeating the same tests. Not only were we concerned that Rick would not be given proven therapies for his condition to assist in his healing, but an incorrect diagnosis could create long-term, residential care issues, possibly affecting his long-term care insurance coverage.

I've included in this chapter some of the emails highlighting important background about his case for perspectives it may offer to others similarly afflicted with underlying toxic issues. In sending these to Rick's psychiatric team, I naively believed they would find the information valuable and begin administering the therapies that would expedite his recovery.

As you will see, the information was met with resistance without exploration of its validity. While I initially viewed this stay as a sanctuary of hope for Rick's recovery, I soon discovered it was mired in the false promise of pharmaceuticals, without any consideration to the underlying causes. Although this correspondence failed to achieve its desired impact upon Rick's treatment, they are provided here for you which may offer new insights and pathways for exploration.

First, they dismissed the QEEQ findings from Dr. D, Rick's friend and former psychologist who wrote:

> "I have been treating bi-polar and brain injured individuals for over 20 years and his presentation upon entering my care in September 2006 through the period up to the date of his arrest was not primary depression let alone bi-polar disorder. He had not during my care manifest the hallmark symptoms of the alleged disorder. Instead, in the opinion of his treating neurologist and his internist, he likely is suffering from "disrupted sleep architecture, possibly bipolar or behavioral issues due to frontotemporal dementia . . .

> "The above constellation of findings, taken together, represent the kind of applied neuroscience finding that constitute the basis for making a diagnosis of an organic disorder rather than a one derived from behaviorally observed psychiatric diagnoses. The DSM-IV manual explicitly rules out the use of the psychiatric diagnosis as primary if there is evidence of an underlying organic disorder. I had argued upon the completion of my QEEG assessment that this man suffered from encephalopathy of unknown origin. During the course of treatment as emotional dysregulation became increasingly apparent, the diagnosis of affective disorder secondary to an organic disorder was added to my clinical diagnosis . . .

> "By that time neurological examinations were documenting symptoms but not ideology. It was for that reason that the QEEG study was recommended. As stated previously that study clearly documented parietal and occipital slowing as well as front left activation. That front left activation is consistent with frontal lobe disconnection syndrome.

Neither of those findings is consistent with a bi-polar condition. Neither dynamic EEG nor QEEG features are construed here as diagnostic for any psychiatric condition, but they do provide converging validity to the conclusions already derived from the medical and psychological assessments that were independently obtained at that time . . ."

September 27

"I am writing to call off the search, to call off the need for more tests. What you are looking for is not currently available—clear, unmistakable evidence, reliable tests that confirm the presence of an organic causes. The *Borrelia* spirochete (note to readers, a spiral pathogen which among many illnesses causes Lyme disease) is like a Stealth bomber—it quietly drops the bomb that destroys both body and brain without its victims even realizing they have been attacked, often without the "bullseye" mark. Yet, that tiny tick will have devastating impact especially for the genetically susceptible. It does not leave many clues, at least those which are accepted and sufficiently peer-reviewed enough at the moment that a clear diagnosis can be given.

The answer as to what has and continues to ravage Rick's body and brain is inflammation caused from multiple toxic causes. Lyme has become an epidemic, and the *Borrelia* spirochete is sweeping deer-infested areas and shattering every aspect of its victims' lives ... their health, relationships, livelihoods, and hope.

We stand at a point in time when evidence is mounting as to the utter destruction this disease causes, yet science is still investigating and discounting its impact. Meanwhile, patients and their loved ones seek answers as to what has caused all this physical, emotional, and mental suffering. Their cases are complex, and they are subjected to an onslaught of tests and repeated tests with the hopes that the mystery will be solved with some EEG tracing, CT scan, MRI, a known virus, or bacteria to point to and finally be relieved that at least they knew they had not just lost their minds. Unfortunately, spirochetes "hide," and tests are unreliable. If it does not show through the Western Blot and ELISA tests, it's typically dismissed.

Ultimately for insurance purposes and to wrap some label around a condition, a patient is given a diagnosis, even if not accurate, that can be explained, squeezed into diagnostic boxes, yet do not really fit. Some patients are subjected to inferences that they are hypochondriacs, because surely a patient cannot have so many changing symptoms! Or perhaps explained as stress-related and that "life just becomes too much" and so prescribed a plethora of drugs to treat anxiety or depression symptoms.

As seems to be the case with this disease and its multiple symptoms, doctors look at the body of "evidence." They filter their evaluations through what is currently known science, with so much more to be learned. Meanwhile, the drugs do not work, and patients' physical pain and anguish is unrelenting.

Yet, some like Dr. Shoemaker who have worked with patients with these mysterious symptoms know we stand at a point in time when much is yet to be revealed. These doctors face ridicule and their brilliant research invalidated or questioned by some, because they recognize there is much to discover. They are willing to step outside the box of an accepted medical framework with hope that their efforts will eliminate suffering and to eliminate this scourge for the future.

So where are we? Rick's vital signs are good, his blood is likely also deceptively within normal range without investigating all the markers indicating a direct link to a toxic-related illness. That is the cruelest part of this disease. Standard tests do not reveal what is happening inside and it's so tragic. I called him yesterday and he can barely speak. This disease is taking him down. My wish if I could have one for him, is to stop the traditional testing because it will not be revealed. Rick's tested positive for Lyme through specific biomarkers and even that is difficult with this stealth-like disease.

Give him drugs to help his pain, for his nerves and to offer comfort, because he is suffering from a medical condition. Time is fleeting. If his condition is not acknowledged for what it is, there is little hope. He will continue to suffer without assistance of therapies that might otherwise make a defining difference. Without being open-minded to ground-breaking research and therapies that are proving to recover health, my husband's future is in jeopardy, as are all the others similarly afflicted."

(Postscript added in 2021): Although the primary culprit of Rick's illness was polytoxicity, toxic poisoning from multiple agents, his high inflammatory markers from previous testing at the CRBAI showed an unquestionable link to CIRS. In addition to his excessively high inflammatory marker of MMP9, Rick's C3d marker was low, now recognized by Lyme literate doctors as another indicator of Lyme. Now, with the evolving research of this dreaded disease, doctors who are not open to new insights or explore such links to a patient's conditions are committing inexplicable care.

**

September 27—Upon receiving communication from his psychiatrist earlier that day refuting claims of Rick's Lyme diagnosis as a contributing factor of neurotoxicity, I drafted this email:

"Rick's sick and getting sicker. I am helpless to do anything more.

Dr. Shoemaker's markers clearly make the point he is dealing with post-Lyme issues, but if these are disputed and not considered 'valid," then, I suppose that's it. There is nothing left as "evidence" except a sick man on Ward A-6 who has markers which are not being validated.

Rick fits the biotoxic model to a "T" with markers way off the charts. It is such a logical pattern and puts all the pieces together as to what made him so sick. Why it is being discredited, I don't understand all the politics.

It is pathogenic, organic and yet science isn't up to speed to validate. Where does that leave us? If you are unwilling to accept the evidence I have provided, then he's slapped with a psychiatric label that's only a symptom of what's underlying all his suffering and relegated to a painful existence? Why are minds so closed? Shouldn't we be asking more questions and considering new realities?

Most of us who have loved ones mysteriously afflicted are not scientists, but we have done plenty of research, and that seems to put "a bee up some bonnets" for some physicians. We are determined to have our loved ones' illnesses validated for what they are and that they are treated accordingly. Although we may be worn down from all the frustration, we are on a passionate quest for science to validate what's ravaging and ruining our loved ones' lives. We feel such despair in this siege of overwhelming invalidation, not to mention lack of help in alleviating their suffering.

It is the dawning of a new era and it is terrifying knowing that invisible things can cause such havoc. Scientists can dispute it, yet toxin-exposed patients and their families are its current victims. This is not just about Rick. I have seen so many who are suffering from toxic-related illnesses. You see, there is a growing community linked together by them. We are united in our frustration of traditional healthcare's inability to evaluate with methods proven in evolving science.

My heart is broken and now even more so because I have nothing left to give you. Medicine does not embrace what it does not fully understand until all the evidence is in. Meanwhile, while the verdict is "out," we are suspended in a world of complete destruction, knowing our loved ones are suffering. No number of antidepressants, anti-psychotics, or anti-anxiety meds will ever resolve it because medications cannot treat the underlying issues.

Then, there is another insult, a financial nightmare regarding insurance which does not cover most of the tests that pinpoint to toxicity. At a time when finances have tightened due to the inability of a partner to work, and often the caregiver, we take on more financial obligations to secure tests and therapies proven to work. We are living in a hell, tortured without the existence of tests accepted by mainstream medicine. Toxic-associated illnesses have wiped out entire families, bank accounts, and bankrupted hearts, not to mention taken lives.

Look at Rick's history, clean slate before, no drugs whatsoever. Nothing … not even a blood pressure pill, cholesterol-reducing pill, or anti-depressant. He did not drink. No midlife crisis. We loved and supported each other. We were a happy family with so many blessings.

Ever since entering the healthcare system 3½ years ago, Rick has had so many chemical cocktails prescribed but nothing has worked, because psychiatric issues are not the cause of manifestation of multiple symptoms. All those drugs have only added to his toxic body burden, and his genetics test proved he is compromised to process them out. Yet, if he is being viewed as a psychiatric patient, it is indeed hopeless, because the true cause of all his symptoms is being dismissed, discredited, or overlooked.

Down the road, all the evidence will be in. Ultimately, what is now termed "late onset bipolar" or "depression" will be recognized for what it is, caused from organic agents, be it a bug bite, mold, a chemical, nutritional imbalances or from something else that disrupts brain function, and not because of your term, "decompensation" or an inability to handle life.

Please note information below regarding the testing. This is EXACTLY the problem and I hope it lands into open minds.

So now what?

1. The Centers for Disease Control and Prevention (CDC) surveillance criteria for Lyme disease were devised to track a narrow band of cases for epidemiologic purposes. As stated on the CDC website, the surveillance criteria were **never** intended to be used as diagnostic criteria, nor were they meant to define the entire scope of Lyme disease.

2. The **ELISA** screening test is unreliable. The test **misses 35%** of culture proven Lyme disease (only 65% sensitivity) and is unacceptable as the first step of a two-step screening protocol. By definition, a screening test should have at least 95% sensitivity.

3. Of patients with acute culture-proven Lyme disease, **20–30% remain seronegative** on serial **Western Blot** sampling. Antibody titers also appear to decline over time; thus, while the Western Blot may remain positive for months, it may not always be sensitive enough to detect chronic infection with the Lyme spirochete. For "epidemiological purposes" the CDC eliminated from the Western Blot analysis the reading of **bands 31 and 34**. These bands are so specific to *Borrelia burgdorferi* that they were chosen for vaccine development. Since a vaccine for Lyme disease is currently unavailable, however, a positive 31 or 34 band is highly indicative of *Borrelia burgdorferi* exposure. Yet these bands are not reported in commercial Lyme tests."

September 29

"A key finding related in Rick's case is his HLA genotype making him especially vulnerable to manifest a chronic illness when triggered by one or more biotoxins. I have already sent his Lyme biomarkers. I am now attaching the mold lab tests revealing several different spores with *Penicillum/aspergillus* as the highest of the seven different varieties in our basement. His upstairs office contained *Cladosporium* and *Penicillium/aspergillus*, as the highest levels of the nine different varieties found.

It seems vital at this point that this biotoxin research is seriously given consideration. From our experience, we have met resistance on numerous occasions from mainstream medicine's refusal to connect Rick's illness to organic causes. I hope your team will be receptive because it offers the potential for transforming his health.

You asked what might help. While I wish it were a matter of adjusting medications and finding the right mix and strength of mood stabilizers, they simply will not resolve all the multiple issues related to this condition.

What Rick really needs is more MSH, a hormone, no longer available, which according to CRBAI research would help to alleviate so much suffering. MSH for biotoxic patients would assist them much like insulin for a diabetic. Rick barely had any MSH from his 2005 test. I urge you to test for his MSH level again as one form of confirmation of his condition.

I request your consideration of the following: 1) that Rick is prescribed the Shoemaker protocol to assist in detoxification and 2) that he is placed back on the nutritional cleansing program I offered to send to the hospital earlier. This is a multi-system cleanse system of organic ingredients which flushes impurities from tissues and was valuable to him in the past. It also provides bioavailable ingredients for nutritional support and helpful in gaining back energy, improving mental clarity, and helping to correct other imbalances.

Rick returned from the nearly dead when he was regularly detoxifying, becoming the most functional since being stricken in spring 2004. However, after he moved out and HIPAA'd me out of his care, Rick abandoned his detoxification protocol, supplements, and healthy diet.

I realize this isn't your typical protocol but without this, he will continue to decline and unable to participate in the planned neuropsych exam. If you provide permission to have Rick on a detoxification program, I will happily work with your nursing staff for implementation.

He has been in obvious and extreme physical distress complaining of severe weakness and difficulty in walking. He seems to have a very hard time getting enough oxygen to speak, likely due to low VEGF which accompanies this condition as explained in information forwarded to you earlier. Might there also be some accommodation in assisting his mobility since this is another source of anxiety in his weakened state?

Rick's case is complex, and I ask for your willingness to consider both his physical and cognitive decline as stemming from organic causes. New pathogens and the illnesses caused by them are now prevalent throughout our healthcare system. Huge knowledge gaps regarding evaluation and treatment are a major missing piece contributing to patient recovery from neurotoxic illnesses.

Blessings to each one of you, for we have been surrounded by a network of willing souls throughout this challenge to carry us through."

***

After all the flurry of documentation of Rick's diverse toxic-related tests validating his inflammatory illness, I received this disheartening response from his treating psychiatrist. It is provided here, illustrating the flagrant dismissal of groundbreaking research data. If it had been accepted, it likely would have changed the course of his treatment and recovery. The psychiatrist tenaciously held to his belief that Rick's issues were of a non-organic nature.

"Dear Mrs. Strauss,

Years ago, I heard a story that went something like this: When someone asked Edison how it felt that so many of his experiments to produce a working light bulb had failed, he exclaimed: "I never failed ... I simply found many ways that did not work; and I got excited every time."

You once believed that the Lyme Test confirmed that Richard had once been infected with Lyme. I spoke with 2 supervisors at LabCorp who stated unequivocally that the lab test in question confirmed the ABSENCE of a previous Lyme infection. Despite this you continue insist that Richard's condition is due to Lyme. Is that logical? An axiom in medicine says: "Adequate treatment is based upon accurate diagnosis." In the past, treatment for Lyme did not help Richard because he NEVER had Lyme. We, like Edison, should be ***excited*** to know that we have proved that he doesn't need THAT treatment.

Richard may still be suffering from an organic process and we need to complete the EEG, MRI and Neuropsychological Testing suggested by Dr. Harrison. I promise that I will not proceed with an LP (lumbar puncture) without discussing it with you and Rick's brother.

Richard's clinical history clearly suggests TREATABLE conditions that do NOT require us to suspend logic or rely on misinterpreted tests or un-proven and un-confirmable data.

One final recommendation (for this email). I have read enough articles about Lyme Disease - so have you. My advice is to stop. On the other hand, I am going to suggest that you re-read some of your own books, articles, and lecture notes. If you believe what you have said and written about the importance of a positive mental attitude, I beg you: live what you have taught. ESPECIALLY IN YOUR INTERACTIONS WITH RICHARD.

My team and I will continue to work to help Richard feel and function better. We have not given up hope and I encourage you to remain positive; and EXPECT him to get better - he may yet surprise you by living UP to those expectations."

Rick's treating psychiatrist, Dr. A

(Name withheld to protect his arrogance!)

***

With his doctor obviously close-minded about Rick's biotoxic exposures, I forwarded documentation regarding Rick's high heavy metals test in hopes that would be recognized as another causal agent of his neurotoxicity:

My response back to Dr. A responding to his email:

October 5

"To provide you with as complete a medical/life history on behalf of Rick, here is his provoked urine toxic tests from 2004. The 24-hour urine collection was authorized by Norman Levin, MD, an internist/rheumatologist. Rick had long-term exposures to chemical solvents, lead-paint/pipes in his early 20th century home, suspected as another inflammatory agent. Additionally, he had several hair samples showing high levels of lead, cadmium, and other toxic metals.

We acknowledge that you are addressing Rick's case with considerable evaluation. In that same vein, by factoring the neurotoxic roots of his condition, then his mental state, pain, weakness, shortness of breath, tremors, insomnia, appetite changes, and other symptoms must be viewed from that perspective as further explanation for his deteriorated condition.

If only Rick's recent history is reviewed and evaluated from a purely psychiatric perspective, then deductions are made with a case built upon psychiatric issues. However, Rick's life up until being slammed at age 59 was a long history of good health and no psychiatric issues or even a therapy session prior to 2004, when multiple symptoms appeared.

Rick's long-term exposure to a multitude of toxic substances, confirmed through lab tests for mold, metals and other markers, along with a genetic marker demonstrating his body's compromised ability to process out toxins, must be taken seriously into consideration as contributing agents of his inflammatory illness.

With a body burden of lifetime exposures to many toxic chemical solvents, high levels of lead, aluminum, manganese, chromium, and other heavy metals, in addition to confirmed long-term exposure to toxic mold and suspected Lyme disease, all combine to create a perilous neurotoxic domino effect.

Please share the metals tests with the team as well as previous biotoxin lab tests. His diagnosis of toxic encephalopathy is valid and may now be further compounded from the deterioration caused by this condition."

October 12

"I do not understand why you continue to dismiss data regarding the environmental impact which has significant bearing upon Rick's deterioration.

Yes, indeed, many of us do have plenty of chemicals, metals, biotoxins and other toxins swirling throughout our bodies which may be precisely the reason why we have such a national health crisis—more cases of many diseases striking at alarming rates, young and old. It does not mean we're safe. It means if you are genetically susceptible, you are more likely to be stricken.

I am not sure why you continue to dismiss or invalidate the CRBAI research that points to Rick's neurotoxic exposure. It appears you want to rule out environmental issues even though they offer valuable clues. I thought scientists revel in new research that might just explain what is happening to their patient's health and follow the trail of the markers that could point the way to a plausible and very possible explanation. History and science are constantly unveiling new answers and disproving long-held theories. Environmental exposure is the new frontier.

I have a large, varied network with many or their loved ones experiencing such a wide range of brain disorders, early onset of dementias and other chronic, debilitating diseases. We live in a new era when we do not know it all quite yet. It is a time to consider that which is yet to be proven does not mean it's not a valid consideration.

As described earlier, the pattern to Rick's illness is in direct congruence to his genetics to develop an inflammatory illness from neurotoxic exposure, so why is this research and data been discredited when he fits the biotoxin profile to a T and beyond? His numbers were off the charts!

If you want to give him a painless, cheap test, give him the VCS test that serves as a good screening device for neurotoxic exposure. Run him through the tests that serve as reliable markers for neurotoxic exposure and look how he stacks up with the neurotoxic profile as described in *Mold Warriors*. As mentioned earlier, the traditional tests you are running will NOT show what is really flaring all his symptoms. They are not the right diagnostic tests for what now ails him and so many others because our world is changing, and our bodies are suffering the consequences. Research that is currently accepted in traditional medicine simply has not caught up with it all … yet.

Environmental exposure for the genetically vulnerable ignites biochemical imbalances with multiple symptoms. They develop chronic fatiguing illnesses and cannot breathe at times with links to respiratory issues. Their brains become inflamed. Their behavior changes and so do their moods. Movement becomes difficult. They grow weak and develop changing symptoms of varying duration and intensity. So, it all makes sense, as well as why the psychotropic therapies are not working because they're not addressing the root causes!

Your September 27 email stated Rick did not have Lyme (according to the results from widely recognized, unreliable tests). Yet, this is precisely at a time when the debate rages on within the medical community because current tests are unreliable. At a time when so many doctors, scientists, and researchers are in obvious disagreement, post-Lyme certainly CANNOT be ruled out, nor Rick's exposure to mold, earlier chemical exposure or from toxic metals. These cannot be dismissed as compounding agents to his decline because enough evidence supports how each of these things ALONE can cause exactly the symptoms Rick has manifested.

As science evolves, the connection of these same root factors will be linked to the mounting epidemics of cancer, obesity, and disorders of every system of the body. Stress is indeed a contributing cause, but so are our genetic predispositions, toxic environmental exposures, nutritional imbalances, and other influences flaring inflammation. We are living in a time exploding with lots of questions as to why we now have life-threatening epidemics, and the explanations/diagnoses are no longer accurate. So, it is with great hope that you seriously consider these factors, as a vital link regarding Rick's treatment, yet with respect to all your current and future patients.

That is why I must advocate for Rick and for others suffering from similar maladies. In my career as a consumer educator, I simply cannot remain silent regarding the resistance to assist patients through proper testing and therapies which can make a difference to their recovery.

Too many lives are being ravaged from this horrific affliction. Science is revealing answers, yet until mainstream medicine embraces revolutionary wisdom, patients will be at the mercy of practitioners holding on to outdated models."

It's a Different Dementia!

November

Rick's psychiatric team repeated the same tests he had undergone in previous years, with similar results. His latest MRI revealed comparable deficits. Now, they wanted to repeat comprehensive neuropsych tests, although I had provided them with the results of his earlier neuropsych testing upon his admission.

The team assigned Rick a PhD post-doctoral fellow in clinical neuropsychology to conduct a fourth series of tests. As earlier testing had indicated, they clearly demonstrated his cognitive decline and behavioral issues, linked to a neurodegenerative disorder diagnosed as subcortical dementia. This is characterized by slowness of mental processing, forgetfulness, impaired cognition, apathy, and depression.

Subcortical dementia differs from the more traditional characteristics of Alzheimer's dementia. It is related to a different part of the brain with cerebral cortical involvement, including memory loss, impairments in reading comprehension and language expression, inability to recognize familiar objects and faces, and others.[1]

This was the summary following Rick's fourth series of neuropsychological testing:

> "Mr. Strauss' performance is consistent with a neurodegenerative disorder, such as a subcortical dementia. Although frontotemporal dementia is also a possibility, his limited decline in memory is inconsistent with that diagnosis. Although he has a history of mood dysfunction and was notably anxious during the testing, it is more likely that his cognitive symptoms preceded his anxiety and mood difficulty (given his reported initial difficulties at work). **Therefore, his mood and anxiety symptoms only exacerbate the symptoms of his neurodegenerative condition."**

At last, we had a definitive diagnosis, which was finally accepted! According to this evaluation, Rick suffered from a more unfamiliar frontal/subcortical dementia, which is strikingly different from the more common and familiar form of Alzheimer's disease in the following ways:

- Affects prefrontal cortex, white matter, basal ganglia, thalamus
- Recent memory often normal or only mildly impaired
- Loss of drive, disinhibition common
- Executive dysfunction common

- MMSE (Mini Mental State Exam) is useless, with results often near-normal

  "In general, these illnesses are not detected with typical bedside screening or with conventional dementia assessment tools, such as the Mini Mental State Exam. These illnesses are associated with prominent and disturbing behavioral changes, as well as difficulties with "higher-order" cognitive functions, such as planning and judgment... Familiarity with this clinical picture is essential for recognition, diagnosis, and management of these illnesses, and for working with families and caregivers."[2]

At my request, Rick's treating psychiatrist reluctantly provided me with these test results because they confirmed that, in fact, his condition was neurodegenerative in nature and not a condition that medications would resolve.

It finally gave legitimacy to the reality of his illness, which I had fought for relentlessly for years. I was also relieved to finally have the documentation needed to qualify for Rick's long-term care insurance, which otherwise might have been denied.

Questions without Answers

Why did all the psychiatrists, even those specializing in geriatrics and memory disorders, overlook these less familiar dementing illnesses and discount neurodegenerative decline? What is especially perplexing is that these dementias were recognized decades earlier in medical journals, as evidenced by the *PubMed* article published in 1984, as referenced in the previous section.

When a patient lands in a psych ward or mental hospital, why would there be so much resistance that a patient's symptoms are related to an organic cause? Or that there are other solutions that exist beyond a cocktail of drugs to correct brain issues?

Had Rick been properly evaluated and treated for the root causes of his chronic inflammation years earlier, what a difference that might have made! It may not have lessened the pain and suffering that naturally comes from loss of faculties and a raging, inflamed body, but it would have eliminated years of heartache and its collateral damage:

- It would have explained how neurotoxicity and brain inflammation had transformed Rick into a stranger. Instead of fueling our anger and fear from his erratic behavior, with a better understanding of his illness we could have tempered our responses with more love and compassion.

- It would have eliminated the need for ECT and toxic drug treatments, which further added to Rick's toxic burden and heightened his inflammatory responses.

- It would have eliminated the need to have Rick arrested to get into a temporary, safe environment for evaluation.

- I would have retained my role as Rick's health advocate every step of the way, instead of being excluded from his care decision during a most critical time, putting his life and others at risk.

- I would have retained my responsibilities as his POA, allowing me to make all financial and legal decisions on his behalf and protecting our financial resources. Instead, while Rick lived unsupervised, he went on wild spending sprees, and I was legally unable to stop him. With the revocation of his POA, I had to seek legal guardianship and conservatorship, resulting in significant legal and accounting fees over the years, adding more burden during a time of excessive stress.

Chapter 11
The Roller Coaster Ride of Cognition and Care
(December 2007-April 2016)

Lockdown in Memory Care

December 2007

In mid-December, after six months of confinement at Virginia's state psychiatric facility in central Virginia, Rick was transferred to Northern Virginia Mental Health Institute in Falls Church, near our home. As Rick's co-guardians, Lowell and I met Rick at the Institute for his case review. It was obvious that neither his cognition nor his demeanor had improved since his admission in the summer.

Based on Rick's recent neuropsych testing, both the care advisor and medical team recommended that Rick reside in a locked dementia unit for his safety. Our next challenge was finding a facility that would accept Rick. Since behavioral issues are often associated with patients having frontal lobe brain issues, several would not consider admitting him for this reason.

Luckily, our care consultant recommended a facility exclusively devoted to dementia patients, which had a room available. The facility closest to our house would not have availability for a while, so for a few months Rick was placed in a sister location, about an hour away (without traffic) in Maryland. The commute proved arduous. I eagerly awaited availability in the neighboring location, closer to our home.

It had been nearly a year since I was able to supervise any facet of Rick's care. I explained to the doctor at the facility that Rick needed to be back on his former nutritional and detoxification regimen. It was such a relief not to battle with either the doctor or the nursing staff to ensure Rick's treatment! Although that alone was one less strain, the long commute to Maryland proved exhausting. Fortunately, within a few months a room became available closer to home, and we transferred Rick to the memory care facility about a 40-minute drive away—closer, but still a long commute especially during rush hour in northern Virginia.

Rick's memory was not too impaired, but he was extremely withdrawn. As time went on, he grew more conversational, but not at all animated. I became increasingly concerned about his social engagement since all residents were about a generation older, most wandering the hallways in their dementia-states. While Rick seemed content just to remain in his room, it bothered me that he was not having much interaction or stimulation, knowing how valuable that is to health.

June 2008

After nearly two years of long drives for visits several times each week, I explored other options closer to home with the potential for Rick's greater social engagement. After visiting several facilities, I selected a Sunrise facility with a memory care unit, just a few miles from home. I had only to wait a short time for an available room; being closer allowed me to visit Rick more frequently.

Gratefully, they included his vital detoxification protocols into his care plan. The difference was dramatic. Another positive point was that staff members really engaged him and encouraged his participation in activities.

Over time, Rick started to connect more with people. He surprised us all with his increasing clarity and a return to his calmer, more charismatic self. Flickers of his wry wit returned. By now, "Wicked Rick" had long disappeared. Despite this, I would never again be lulled into thinking that I could ever bring him home; his doctor concurred. For his safety and the safety of others, Rick would always require round-the-clock supervision.

Heart Reflections

With Rick's care issues resolved and now residing in a facility best suited to his needs, my life became less strenuous, at least for a time. I finally took the time to reflect on how this arduous journey had changed me and the need to reconstruct my life now that Rick and I would forever be living apart. For years, my own unmet needs had been put on hold while looking after Rick's and my mom's. I sought spiritual counsel from our friend, Lowell, who always provided me with the right guidance both before and throughout the journey of Rick's illness.

Lowell echoed what had been rising within my heart: that the very nature of Rick's illness had shattered our respective roles in marriage, but not our deep love for one another. While our relationship would be forever changed, the bonds of our love could never be broken. I was forever destined to ensure his well-being.

I greatly trusted Lowell's spiritual guidance, both before and throughout this journey with Rick. As his guardian, I would continue to love and support Rick and arrange for the best care suited to his needs. Lowell also counseled me that it was time to move forward with my own life in ways that called to my soul. I continued to search my heart for direction in creating a new life when the one I had expected to evolve had shattered into tiny pieces.

Making a Comeback!

2009

More than a year after moving Rick into the memory care unit at Sunrise, his condition dramatically improved. I attributed this to the continuation of his detoxification and supplement regimen, coupled with the Shoemaker protocol for removing biotoxins.

The admissions manager recommended that Rick be moved back into a regular assisted living unit. Admittedly, I was initially concerned if this was the right move but agreed to their suggestion. Although the administrators did not think Rick would be a flight risk, they initially fitted him with an ankle alarm in case he wandered out the door.

While that turned out to be a very positive move, it still bothered Lowell and me that Rick languished on his bed, isolated for most of the day except mealtimes. We both recognized the importance of service and helping others by sharing our gifts and time. During our visits and calls, we both urged Rick to find some ways to serve.

Over time, Rick seemed to awaken and plug back into life. He began pushing people in their wheelchairs, making kind and loving remarks to caregivers, residents and their visitors, and others. He took on the responsibility of walking the resident Sunrise dog and became quite attached to him. Eventually, Rick was so engaged in the community with his welcoming demeanor and humor that he gained the unofficial title of "The Mayor of Sunrise."

Rick participated in resident meetings and established friendships. During their 2010 holiday party, the social director gave him a leading role in *The Christmas Carol* program. Watching Rick in the starring role, I wiped away tears as he read his lines flawlessly. Beaming with pride, I turned to the woman seated next to me and exclaimed, "If you only had seen him a year ago! What a miracle!"

That evening, Rick received a shiny, gold cardboard star with his name in the middle. That star would hang proudly in all his subsequent rooms from that day forward.

Face-to-Face with Another Inflammatory Reaction

July 2010

I received a call from Sunrise prior to their July 4 celebration. Rick had developed Bell's Palsy and they wanted to alert me prior to my visit. Bell's Palsy can cause a temporary or permanent weakness in facial muscles, resulting in a one-sided smile and a "lazy eye." The doctor did his best to reassure me that the condition was likely temporary, which proved to be true for Rick.

I researched to learn more about Bell's Palsy. Those stricken usually begin to get better within two weeks after the onset of symptoms, with most recovering completely within three to six months.[1] The condition is the result of inflammation of the seventh cranial nerve that runs between the brain and face, exerting pressure on a small gap in the skull. This wears away the protective sheath covering the nerve, causing part of the face to droop, inability to close an eye, slurred speech, tearing, and facial pain.

Cranial neuritis—inflammation of the cranial nerves, which can manifest as Bell's Palsy—double vision and optic neuritis are experienced by about a quarter of Lyme patients. The presence of the Epstein-Barr virus (EBV) is the suspected cause of Bell's Palsy. Epstein-Barr is also the virus linked to mononucleosis; Rick had a confirmed case of mono in his early 20s.

I was grateful that staff had prepared me, because otherwise I might have assumed Rick had suffered a stroke when I saw his one-sided, droopy face. Besides his alarming facial appearance, the palsy caused his eye to tear. Rick was fitted with an eye patch, a "disguise" he turned into humorous "pirate" references, to the amusement of the staff and residents.

September-December

Stacy and Jesse had been in a long-term relationship since their senior year at Virginia Tech. Upon his return from his army tour in Afghanistan, he proposed to her, and they were engaged in September. An engagement party was planned in December. In preparation, since Rick had regained a desire for good grooming habits, he wanted to shed some pounds (he was now close to 300) and more seriously commit to his goals using the same cleansing and fat-burning system that had been so transformative in the past.

I reviewed the instructions with the nursing staff to help him achieve his goals. They were surprised to see Rick not only lose 25 pounds in a few months, but also become much more aware and animated. His results were in alignment with many others on that program who reported feeling more focused and energetic while achieving their weight loss goals.

When I told Rick that I would bring some new clothes to fit his trimmed physique, he expressed eagerness to attend the engagement party in our home. However, when that day arrived, he called to tell me he did not feel well enough to attend. It was another disappointment for all of us, and especially for Stacy, who wanted her Daddy to be part of their celebration.

A Walk Down the Aisle and a Daddy-Daughter Dance

May 2011

Rick had missed many special occasions since the onset of his illness seven years earlier, including Stacy's high school graduation, Stephanie's and Stacy's college graduations, and Stacy's engagement party. Now that his condition had continued to improve, he wanted to participate in Stacy's wedding celebration. Stacy insisted that her father walk her down the aisle. Rick had come a long way, and this walk down the aisle was something to celebrate—symbolic of all our family had come through.

Indeed, when he and Stacy walked down the aisle with dignity and pride, I silently blessed every step he took. They met me halfway, and the three of us linked arms and walked together to the altar. When Rick kissed Stacy on the cheek to give her away, tears welled up in my eyes, and in the eyes of other guests who knew our family's journey and the significance of this moment. Weddings are whirlwinds of rapid-fire precious moments, and to our delight, Rick graced every one of them.

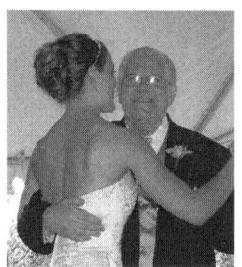

At the reception, Stacy and her dad took to the dance floor for the traditional father-daughter dance. I cried again seeing Rick as a proud papa, dancing with his daughter and remembering the countless moments he had missed over the last seven years. It was a moment captured in his and many hearts because it was also a celebration of Rick's indomitable spirit; it was a dance of courage and determination.

Carolina Calling

July 2012

With Stephanie living in California and Stacy now married and residing in South Carolina, there was no need to continue living in the suburban Northern Virginia neighborhood where the girls grew up. With a career as a work and wellness coach, I could work from anywhere.

In 2011, I met Larry who was experiencing a parallel reality: his ex-wife was being treated for metastatic cancer. We both shared a mutual desire to provide support to our loved ones despite a shift in our respective relationships. Larry and I were drawn together at a time when we both needed the nurturing of another person to revive our flagging spirits with a desire to experience joy.

Larry was ready to retire soon and had an eye on the country life. With Stacy's announcement that she and Jesse were planning to raise their family in the Carolinas, the idea of moving there took root. I was also looking for ways to stretch Rick's long-term care benefits because expenses in northern Virginia were quite high. Rick loved the Sunrise facility in Virginia, and I learned we could save significantly on Rick's care at a similar Sunrise facility in Charlotte, North Carolina.

Although my responsibilities for care continued, I had caught Larry's vision of a more serene life. We searched online for a small farm in the Charlotte area, ideally close to the Sunrise care facility where we hoped to transition Rick. Larry and I found a small farm in need of beautification across the border in South Carolina, about 30 miles away. It was not the most convenient choice, but since it was impossible to find the two in close proximity, it offered the best solution for our budget.

After getting things settled at the farm, we moved Rick into a beautiful room overlooking a tranquil pond at Sunrise. The transition seemed to work perfectly for Rick, who connected easily with several residents and stepped up to be of service—once again assisting residents in wheelchairs while passing along compliments and kindnesses to residents, staff, and visitors. I continued our regular visits, taking him out for lunches, dinners, and doctor's appointments.

The adventures of farm life, along with the animals that soon populated our farm, were soothing balms for our stressed-out souls. A few months later, with visits from both our sisters who had recently attended barn weddings, independently suggested that our farm would be ideal as a rustic wedding venue. That never-imagined idea struck a chord within our creative spirits!

We consulted with several wedding professionals, who all echoed the venue possibilities on our property. So, we began the magical transformation of a flowerless farm into a beautiful space for celebrating love, creating a wedding venue as a joint business venture. Neither of us knew anything about the wedding business, but we both harnessed our respective, complementary talents and forged ahead into our new adventure.

January 2013

I received a call from Sunrise that Rick had fallen and was being taken to the emergency room. He had injured his back and was in excruciating pain. Rick was fitted with a very uncomfortable brace that he hated wearing, and now required a wheelchair. He was placed in a rehab center for about two months in hopes his pain would lessen and his movement improve. Unfortunately, it did not help. Although I brought everything Rick needed to continue his nutritional and detoxification regimen, the rehab facility did not administer it consistently.

Since Stacy's wedding, Rick had lost all enthusiasm for losing weight and ballooned back up to 360 pounds, restricting his movements. The prescribed physical therapy wasn't getting results so after two months, he was transferred back to Sunrise in Charlotte. Rick now faced the possibility of back surgery.

Fortunately, the surgeon recommended a relatively non-invasive surgery that provides almost instantaneous relief and eliminated the need for the brace. It succeeded and Rick graduated to a walker and no longer needed the constricting, upper body brace. He seemed to literally get back on his feet ... for a time. I firmly reminded him that from now on, he always had to use his walker.

June

Stephanie was disappointed with her career options in LA, and Larry and I suggested she move to the Carolinas and explore employment in the Charlotte area. That idea struck a chord in her and she soon took up residence in a rustic-appointed apartment in our barn loft—perfect for her privacy and providing space for charting new directions. The farm became a sanctuary for our family, nurtured by nature, animals and hosting celebrations of love and other events focused on spiritual exploration.

With Stephanie living on our farm and Stacy and Jesse now just a few hours away in Charleston, provided valuable, frequent family connections for Rick, too.

October

In October, Sunrise went through a thorough renovation that included stripping off wallpaper, painting, and installing new carpet. I received a call late one evening that Rick's behavior had become quite contentious. I suspected that chemical sensitivity or being chemically overburdened with toxic fumes from those renovations had re-ignited a brief spell of aggression, which had been dormant since 2007. I realized it was time to explore options closer to our home in South Carolina for convenience to care, especially in such emergencies, and closer supervision of Rick's health.

Care Closer to Home

December 2014

In early December, I moved Rick into a smaller assisted living facility, about 30 minutes closer, making it easier to visit him more often. Since we moved him from a facility in North Carolina to one in South Carolina, that meant Rick's Medicare arrangements changed, necessitating the choice of new specialists for his care.

I scheduled an appointment with a new neurologist and provided her with Rick's lengthy medical history. She suggested that his tremors might be related to Parkinson's disease (PD). While PD had been considered as a possible diagnosis by earlier physicians, Rick was not characteristic, so it was ruled out. However, more recently, Rick was manifesting more Parkinsonian symptoms, including tremors and balance issues.

His new neurologist suggested a one-month trial of Sinemet, and I agreed, hoping it would help with Rick's symptoms. When it failed to help, the doctor discontinued the drug. That was a good thing, since I would later learn from Mayo Clinic research that this type of drug may actually worsen confusion, hallucinations, and delusions for those with Lewy body dementia,[2] the disease Rick would be diagnosed with only a month later.

A few days after Christmas, I bought Rick an extra wide rollator—a walker with wheels for easier navigating, since movement was challenging. Eager to show him how much easier he could get around, I stopped to visit him. When I entered his room, I found him moaning, face down on the floor next to his bed. Rick had fallen again. Due to the facility rules, even without signs of injury, he was required to go to the ER. He was released without any detectable issues, but a few days later, he fell again, became extremely disoriented, and was again admitted to the hospital. There Rick was diagnosed with a urinary tract infection and given intravenous antibiotic treatment; he became hallucinatory, confusing the nurses with our daughters.

Because Rick had become a fall risk, he could not return to the assisted living facility where we had moved him just weeks earlier. Only skilled nursing facilities are authorized to use a hydraulic lift to assist in cases like Rick's. So, after his discharge, we transferred him to a skilled nursing facility for physical therapy. The admissions director advised me that when his therapy ended, he would either be converted into a long-term resident there or transferred to another skilled nursing facility. Once again, I searched for a new facility close to home that met the criteria for Rick's continued care.

There were no beds available in the facilities that I preferred, so Rick had to remain in the skilled nursing facility until other options became available. While it was clean, I felt Rick was not getting the professional, compassionate care or enriching social interactions. Their meals were unpalatable too. Rick was now losing weight, most of it attributable to the colorless preparation of largely starchy, sugary institutional food. I voiced my concern to the administrator, who sent their dietitian to hear to my concerns while Rick was eating his lunch—a plate filled with brownish foods: battered chicken, batter-fried brown broccoli bits, and a whole, unopened brown sweet potato. I knew I was wasting my breath.

With nutrition so vital to health, hospitals, skilled nursing centers, and all institutions dedicated to wellness should focus on foods that nourish bodies and brains instead of just satisfying calorie requirements or special diets. (As I later discuss in chapter 16, "Gut Issues—Ground Zero for Inflammation," the foods we eat, and the nutrition derived from them are instrumental to supporting a healthy, gut-brain connection.) However, it wasn't just the food at this facility that concerned me. I wanted to find a more suitable place for his needs.

His Dementia Has a New Name

January 2015

Rick's post-hospital follow-up required me to schedule an appointment with the neurologist who had treated him in the hospital. I sat dumbfounded when I heard the neurologist's assessment: "Rick is in the latter stages of Lewy body dementia."

Finally, after eleven years of consultations with geriatric specialists, psychiatrists, neurologists, and psychologists, Rick had a diagnosis recognized by other mainstream health professionals. Although I had come across LBD years before in my research, when I approached his earlier doctors with it as a possibility, my findings were dismissed out of hand.

Now with it being more recognized, LBD is like having a combination diagnosis of Alzheimer's, Parkinson's, and schizophrenia, a triple whammy of symptoms causing so much misery for the patient and challenges for caregivers. Confusion, hallucinations, movement issues, and behavioral problems are all typical with LBD. This perfectly reflected the manifestations of Rick's illness.

What are Lewy bodies? Research has identified the presence of abnormal structures, called Lewy bodies in the brains of people suffering from LBD. As they build up, they keep the brain from producing the right amounts of two critical chemicals: 1) acetylcholine, which affects memory and learning; and 2) dopamine, which affects movement, mood, and sleep. (For more information about LBD characteristics see Appendix D: "Common Symptoms of Lewy Body Dementia.")

Proper diagnosis is critical because if patients are prescribed incorrect medications, complications can occur. LBD shares both pathological and clinical features with Alzheimer's, as well as Parkinson's disease. (For more information about the differences between LBD and Alzheimer's, see Appendix E).

As Dr. James Ellison of the Alzheimer's research group, BrightFocus Foundation, notes:

"Physicians see a response to these antipsychotic medications in LBD that is toxic and even dangerous, similar to the reaction that a person with Parkinson's disease might have to antipsychotic medications. The person with LBD who receives even a small dose of an antipsychotic medication can become profoundly stiff, sedated, and more confused and agitated … In the case of LBD, knowing the diagnosis is of great value, because it may alert clinicians to the potentially hazardous effects that might be produced in LBD patients by antipsychotics, a class of medications still often used (despite recognition of their limited benefits and potential adverse effects) to treat behavioral disturbances in AD. For this reason, even if for no others, identifying LBD is already a very worthwhile endeavor."[3]

The Possibility of Polypharmacy

Unfortunately, eleven years into the disease process, Rick had been prescribed a potent mixture of chemical cocktails, including different antipsychotics. It was impossible to determine if his symptoms were related to the disease or exacerbated by his cocktail of medications.[4] Since the onset of his illness, he had been on so many different combinations of drugs over the years, his conditions had possibly been worsened from "polypharmacy." This is an elusive definition often referencing patients being prescribed too many medications, or when the drugs have been prescribed by many doctors and not well coordinated.[5]

As detailed in a *Toxicology International* feature, "Polypharmacy is sometimes overlooked because the symptoms it causes can be confused with symptoms of normal aging or another disease. Sometime resulting in still more drugs being prescribed to tract [treat] the new symptoms. Some signs that are caused by interactions between drugs or side-effects of drugs can include:

- Tiredness, sleepiness, or decreased alertness

- Constipation, diarrhea, or incontinence

- Loss of appetite

- Confusion (all the time or sometimes)

- Falls

- Depression or lack of interest in usual activities

- Weakness

- Tremor

- Hallucinations—seeing or hearing things

- Anxiety or excitability

- Feeling dizzy

- Decreased sexual behavior

- Skin rashes."[6]

Reviewing this list certainly captures many of the symptoms Rick experienced! As noted in that same study, this condition can result from "extended duration of use of medications that were intended to be used for a limited time. Some medications, prescribed initially for a limited time, become unnecessary and therefore inappropriate if taken for long term."[7]

Rick was given daily pharmaceutical cocktails for a dozen years, and a likely candidate for multiple drug intake (MDI), due to the simultaneous use of prescription and over-the-counter combinations. The fact remains, with his genetics as a poor detoxifier, coupled with confirmation of his body burden of toxins from multiple sources, the impact from all the medications he ingested over all those years raises even more concerns.

Changing Care Challenges

March-August 2015

The neurologist who provided Rick's LBD diagnosis had explained to me that moving people with dementia from place to place often creates setbacks, and patients often do not recover well. No doctor who had previously treated Rick had mentioned this to me. I had moved Rick from an assisted living facility in December, then to a hospital after a fall, and now he resided in a less-than-desirable skilled nursing facility.

I happened to run into Ms. J., the admissions director of the assisted living facility where I had previously hoped to move Rick. I shared with her that as Rick's health was failing again, I was not sure of his life expectancy. She adamantly stated, "Even if he's only there for two weeks, get him out of here!" She promised she would make some calls.

Throughout this journey, we had been blessed with many people who "showed up" to guide us through; Ms. J. was part of that ever-expanding list. Fortunately, a semi-private room had just become available at a skilled nursing facility in Rock Hill, one on the top of my list, and I moved Rick there within days.

What a contrast in the care and services! We arrived at the facility around lunchtime and shortly after settling in, they offered Rick a selection of lunch choices. Choices! His lunch tray contained a colorful fresh fruit salad of pineapple, melon, and blueberries, and a delicious-looking egg salad sandwich. The entire staff at the Rock Hill facility was attentive and caring. I was relieved knowing Rick was now going to get the care he deserved.

A Welcome Rebound

In this new facility, Rick was able to resume his daily detoxification routine and supplements. Again, his cognitive abilities improved. When my sister and brother-in-law visited him in July of 2015, they were shocked at Rick's dramatically improved conversational skills, animation, and overall interaction from the last time they had visited him.

I would later discover that LBD patients experience periods of fluctuating cognition, exhibiting apparent improvement, interspersed with periods of decline. I wished I had known about this when the disease first manifested because it would have explained Rick's characteristic, unpredictable behaviors throughout his illness.

This is unique to LBD because other dementias have a more continuous decline. LBD patients can rebound for relatively short periods, sometimes a few hours, a few days, or even months. This is what makes this disease so confusing because of its erratic nature, and even more puzzling if you are unaware of this distinctive characteristic.

Another perplexing behavior associated with LBD is the fluctuating nature of abilities expressing as "Showtime." This might manifest when they visit with loved ones, friends, during doctor visits, or some special event. Rick exhibited "showtime" behavior on countless occasions, e.g., during Connie and Tim's visit, doctors' visits, or the weekend of Stacy and Jesse's wedding). If friends and family are unfamiliar with this characteristic, it can be troubling for caregivers because "showtime" is so deceiving.

However, since Rick's illness was not diagnosed as LBD until the eleventh year, that made for plenty of crazymaking times. Now it all makes sense.

Why does this happen? It's theorized it may be due to the possible re-routing of neural impulses around a non-functioning part of the brain, allowing some periods of improvement. However, as the disease progresses, there are fewer pathways for the nerve impulses to travel and fewer periods of improvement which last for shorter periods of time.[8]

Although Rick's schmoozing skills had completely disappeared at the onset of his illness, his characteristically charming ways periodically resurfaced for varying lengths of time. Those were treasured times witnessing his joy and offered slices of time when his true essence shined forth.

September-December

Back then, I was unfamiliar with LBD's fluctuating trait of abilities. Neither Rick's neurologist, staff nurses, or others advised me of this attribute. Had I known I would have made other choices regarding his care in the months that followed.

By September, Rick's condition had improved so much that skilled nursing no longer seemed appropriate. His days consisted of either lying in his bed or sitting in the communal space with droopy-headed residents, watching old cowboy movies or sitcoms from earlier eras. Rick's roommate had severe Parkinson's and was uncommunicative and confined to his bed.

Given this, I felt compelled to move him back into assisted living where he would receive more stimulation and vital social interaction. I wanted to give him a more interactive environment, despite the earlier warnings about permanent relapses in dementia patients who are moved from place to place.

I contacted the same assisted living facility that I had visited and liked a year earlier, but they had no rooms available. In anticipation that one would open up soon, their admissions director and nurse evaluated Rick. From their evaluation, they believed he only needed the first-tier level of care! A few weeks later, the director called with good news. Once again, I moved Rick to a new facility.

Rick was able to navigate the halls to the dining room with his walker and now had plenty of alert residents and activities to provide stimulation. The staff was engaging and made Rick feel valued and appreciated. However, the following month Rick's care level escalated to the next tier. Unable to use his walker, he had to use a wheelchair. His hallucinations returned and he required increasing care for activities of daily living—toileting, bathing, and transferring.

Rick's resurrected conversational skills largely disappeared. By the end of December, the staff determined they could no longer manage his care. I was told that he needed to be transferred back to skilled nursing and they recommended hospice care. Hospice care! How could Rick have gone so quickly from overall good functioning just month earlier, to needing hospice care?

Unfortunately, I could see that his neurologist's warnings from the previous year were right on target—dementia patients often suffer from such moves. My desire to offer Rick a more stimulating life likely was more detrimental. I regretted that in trying to provide him the best care, I may have miscalculated his needs. The roller coaster ride of highs and lows which had been so characteristic throughout the twelve years of Rick's illness, now seemed headed to a place without rebounds.

The Last Move

January-April 2016

The room at the skilled nursing center where Rick had resided just a few months earlier was still available. Once again, I packed up his few belongings and moved him back to skilled nursing. The nursing staff remembered his charming ways and gave him a warm welcome. His former roommate with Parkinson's disease had died in the interim. Rick's new roommate was an amicable priest with dementia. Now, Rick was the one who was barely conversational.

His days were mostly spent in bed or a Geri chair, a reclining wheelchair that offers greater comfort during the day. He was no longer able to get in or out of bed alone and had become a major fall risk. Since Rick was obese, the nursing staff had to use a Hoyer hydraulic lift to transfer him safely between his bed and the Geri chair—an undignified but necessary maneuver he had to endure multiple times a day.

Rick's advancing dementia made it impossible for him to use a cellphone, so calls were now made through the nurses' station. However, during my visits, I regularly used FaceTime to call our daughters as well as our good friend, Lowell, who had provided us both with wise counsel, insights, and unconditional love throughout Rick's prolonged illness.

By late February, our daughter, Stacy, was 8 1/2 months pregnant with our grandson, with an expected delivery date of mid-March. By the end of February, the hospice nurse shared with us that Rick was now showing all the traditional signs of impending death. In preparation, Stephanie, Stacy, and Jesse came to visit, surrounding Rick with love and to share some of their memories. Stacy told her dad they were having a son. Rick had few words to share except to repeatedly exclaim, "I love my grandson! I love my grandson!"

By early March, the hospice nurse told me Rick's death seemed imminent. Yet, Rick rallied from the grips of death, surprising even the hospice team. We all believed he was holding out from sheer will to see his grandson before he left Earth. This was eerily reminiscent of the lyrics of one of our favorite songs from the jazz-rock band, Blood, Sweat and Tears: "And when I die and when I'm gone, there'll be one child born in a world to carry on."

Hospice kept me regularly updated. Logan was born on March 14, 2016, and Rick was able meet his grandson later that day via Facetime. Still not very conversant, Rick again repeated in a rather exuberant way, "I love my grandson! I love my grandson!"

On April 8, around 11:00 p.m., an hour before our 39th wedding anniversary, I received a call from the nursing center that Rick had fallen and hit his head. Instead of following hospice instructions that nurses were to contact them in case of emergency, the nurse on duty called for an ambulance and Rick was transported to the hospital. She then called me after the ambulance had taken him there. I immediately called the ER to alert them that Rick was a hospice patient and did not require imaging studies; but it was too late—Rick was already undergoing a CT scan.

I was furious because the last thing I wanted for Rick was for him to undergo one more medical test during his last few days. When I visited him the next morning at the nursing center, the butterfly bandage on his forehead served as a sad reminder of the mishaps from the earlier evening. After all he had endured throughout the dozen years of his illness, my desire was for him to "go quietly into the goodnight." Instead, Rick got another ambulance ride with sirens blaring and more unnecessary tests.

Chapter 12
Making Peace from Our Journey

In his final days, Rick's ability to communicate was negligible as he drifted in and out of consciousness. As I sat at his bedside, he struggled for the words he quietly whispered, repeating over and over, "I love you ... I love you ... I love you." Love was indeed at the heart of our souls' journey together. It gave me the sustenance to keep digging for answers when none were forthcoming because I knew there was much to be discovered. From knowing his loving essence, for a sliver of time buried beneath the many disguises of his illness, we both experienced the heartaches arising from a body and brain on fire.

In the final stages of his life, it was the memory of love and appreciation Rick wished to leave behind. With the confusion, suffering, and heartbreak his illness had provoked, I believe Rick intuitively knew that I always made my decisions throughout the years for his well-being. It had proven to be a time of endurance for both of us and perhaps a perfect reflection of our endearing love.

On April 20, 2016, at age 71, Rick made his transition, finally released from his long siege of suffering. In retrospect, I wish I had requested an autopsy or donated his brain for research—I believe Rick would have approved of one more opportunity to pay it forward. At the time, I just wanted Rick fully released from any more probing of his physical body, even in death.

His memorial service followed a few weeks later. It was fitting that Reverend Lowell, who had played such a vital role in our lives, offered the eulogy. It was a tribute to Rick's love, the many lives he influenced, and the lessons he shared both before and during the latter part of his illness.

During my tribute, I shared a significant lesson I learned from our journey for anyone who ever serves as a caregiver, especially for those who are neuro-logically impaired:

> "You can find yourself forgetting who they were because the person you're now caring for is but a shadow of their former self. It's hard not to yearn for those earlier days because you miss that connection of knowing everything about them, and the tapestry of life you've woven together. This dreadful disease rewires a brain in such a way that there is barely a trace of anything recognizable.
>
> As a caregiver, you are called into service in ways you never imagined— an endurance run of the heart. It is so important to reflect upon their true essence of love, always there but disguised with strange, uncharacteristic

behaviors. Now, it's you who must remember who they were before the disease stole them from you.

Pull out the photos or other mementos to remember all the good things about your relationship, of what you were to one another, of what you will forever cherish that endeared them to you. And lest you forget, because you will at times... their soul, as well as yours, somehow needed to be part of this journey."

Looking Back and Within

Through the blessing of time, I can look back on the tragic consequences of Rick's neurological nightmare with a different perspective. His illness, and millions of other cases, cannot be resolved with 20th century medicine in an age of 21st century health issues.

When Rick's conventional treatment teams were unable to offer plausible insights into his illness, they attempted to manage his symptoms with medications by doling out trial upon trial of pharmaceuticals. The doctors hoped to alter his behavior and symptoms, yet none ever provided that. Yet, most of them were confident that Rick's issues were psychiatric in nature. How many patients, past, present, and future might also be solely evaluated from this limited perspective and thus given medications that do not address what underlies all the symptoms?

Following the early months of testing and evaluation that produced no answers, only by a stroke of good fortune did we find our way to Dr. Shoemaker. He had transformed his family practice into one focused on research and evaluating and treating patients suffering from biotoxic exposures. After we spent a year searching for answers, he was the first medical doctor who ordered tests for specific inflammatory markers. He recognized toxicity for its ability to ignite inflammation wreaking multiple symptoms and imbalances.

What still angers me is that so many doctors would not even consider exploring Dr. Shoemaker's research, which would have confirmed the underlying reasons for Rick's illness. This would have provided proven therapies to help Rick recover. Only Dr. T., an open-minded internist, was willing to delve into unfamiliar science with unfamiliar protocols, offered us welcome support. However, when Dr. T. was diagnosed with cancer, he closed his practice and left us without a local physician who would willingly explore Rick's complex case with equal tenacity.

What a difference it would have made had the other allopathic doctors been intrigued or inspired enough to call Dr. Shoemaker and learn of the significance of Rick's biomarkers and the research presented to them. It seemed they each had their minds made up about his diagnosis based on their observable behaviors, choosing not to factor in anything that was not within the realm of their training.

Until learning of Rick's genetics and environmental exposures, I relied on mainstream medicine's mindset. That is, until it became clear that Rick's care must also include the detoxification therapies recommended. However, due to his psychiatric abnormalities he had to be placed under round-the-clock, supervised care, and monitored by conventional specialists. This all meant sometimes ignoring my desires.

At the time, I was unaware of "functional medicine" as a new approach for evaluating and treating the root causes of inflammation and the resulting cascade of debilitating conditions it can cause. At the time, this new medical model was still in its infancy stages, and I did not discover its existence until after Rick's death. This meant I had to rely on more accessible, traditionally prescribed care available through insurance coverage. However, conventional practices failed to properly diagnose and treat Rick's underlying problems. We were caught between medical models and some uncompromising physicians. Rick was unable to receive the essential detoxification therapies needed for his toxic brain issues. This was especially true as a resident in some long-term care facilities which relied on medications for behavior management.

Upon Rick's official diagnosis with dementia in the fall of 2007, I eventually accepted conventional medicine's belief that Rick's neurological condition was irreversible. Yet, his dementia had been linked to his genetics as a poor detoxifier with a lifetime of toxic exposures, so by continuing the protocols that had shown such promise, I envisioned his transformation. They had proven to dramatically improve his condition, resolve many symptoms and enhance his overall wellbeing.

I held to the belief that no condition, diagnosis, or prognosis is necessarily permanent. Indeed, miracles had appeared along the way, filling me with hope. Other times, I felt despair, with so many unknowns clouding my optimism. Then, waves of guilt would sometimes arise despite me knowing full well that negative thoughts have no place on the pathway of healing. But they arose anyway, entangled with regret, anger, sorrow, and grief when overcome by feelings of helplessness—natural companions as a witness to the pain and debilitation of a loved one.

Since his complex case did not seem to have much of a precedent in medical circles, my optimism was eventually replaced with resignation—that his health destiny was beyond my control. With Rick's diagnosis of what was considered a permanent condition, his care was managed by visiting doctors to facilities where he resided, as well as by me taking him to specialists' offices for continuing assessments. How I wish I would have discovered earlier the emerging functional medical model that held great promise for possibly recovering his health.

Had I known then about functional practitioners with their systems-oriented model of evaluation and treatment to address the underlying causes of disease, and how genetics, lifestyle choices, and environmental exposures all play a role, Rick's entire journey of evaluation and treatment would have been considerably different. He would have been evaluated from the perspective of knowledge of all these interactions with personalized treatments.

Until recently, dementia has been viewed as irreversible, decimating lives with that dreaded diagnosis. Now, by addressing root causes with proven therapeutic interventions that can both prevent and help to recover cognitive decline, health destinies are dramatically changing! Patients who have participated in these life-transforming protocols are experiencing miraculous results as featured in *The First Survivors of Alzheimer's,* released just prior to publication of this book. While Rick's detoxification protocol produced significant improvements, he did not have the benefit of the full range of interventions that are now recognized as critical to recovery. This science-based approach, highlighted in chapter 19, now offers a proven pathway for embracing optimism with solutions beyond hope.

While I did not have the full picture back then, the parts of the puzzle that came together helped me in better understanding his illness and why detoxification and nutritional support were so critical. With Rick's genes and the firestorm those toxins created without receiving proper evaluation or treatment, time was a critical factor. His raging inflammation had caused so many imbalances for too long, that worked against his full recovery.

These questions haunted me throughout the 12-year journey of Rick's illness:

1. Have I done everything to support his healing?

2. Is his condition now beyond an ability to restore his health?

3. Am I projecting my desire for him to heal or am I interfering with a desire he may have to be released from the relentless torment of his inflamed body?

Ultimately, I find comfort in knowing I did my best to untangle the mystery while tenaciously searching for the truth. When the unexpected whirled us into the unknown, I sought solutions, asked for guidance, accepted help, and found great comfort in my connections with caring souls and open-minded practitioners. I gained lessons on a deeper level. I had to let go of expectations of the way life "should be" and accepted "what is" with as much grace and strength as I could muster.

I learned a new dance, moving to a rhythm I would not have chosen. My hope is that I can bring purpose to that long journey by sharing the discoveries I learned along the way that revealed new possibilities.

The following year I learned of revolutionary research that now offers science-based solutions for those with similar neurological issues. Hope was no longer on the horizon, but it had arrived with proven protocols! Patients with poor detoxifying genes, exposed to toxins, and manifesting symptoms similar to Rick's, could now envision a more hopeful future.

Posthumous Postscript: A Groundbreaking Revelation

Alzheimer's disease can be prevented, and in many cases
its associated cognitive decline can be reversed.[1]

Dale E. Bredesen, MD

In September 2017, about 17 months after Rick's death, I listened for the first-time to *The People's Pharmacy*[2] podcast, featuring a segment with Dale E. Bredesen, MD, author of *The End of Alzheimer's—The First Program to Prevent and Reverse Cognitive Decline*.

Dr. Bredesen detailed the evolving research, diagnostic testing, and treatment of Alzheimer's disease through functional evaluation. Yes! The research revealed Alzheimer's is not one condition as often treated, but three subtypes, each with distinctive characteristics. When he mentioned that Type 3 was associated with toxic exposure, genetic predisposition, and other factors, I knew more answers would be revealed.

As soon as the book arrived, I turned to the characteristics of Type 3, and found the details mirroring the exact characteristics and tests associated with Rick's neurological condition. At last! There it was—a comprehensive collection of the common traits, symptoms, and biochemical markers as Rick had experienced. It was a validation of all the data I had compiled in the search for answers throughout his devastating disease. It served as posthumous proof that toxicity from biotoxins, heavy metals, infections, and shortage of supportive nutrients ignited Rick's inflammation.

Bredesen's research team discovered that toxic Type 3 patients are genetically prone to be poor detoxifiers, which triggers the cascade of autoimmune responses and biochemical assaults on the body and brain from inflammation. Rick's neuropsych testing in 2007 pointed to frontotemporal dementia, which was also mentioned in Bredesen's research of Type 3 patients. As Bredesen notes, "Patients with this subtype 3 are often diagnosed initially with something other than Alzheimer's disease, such as frontotemporal dementia or depression, or diagnosed as "atypical Alzheimer's."[3] Rick had been similarly labeled.

To refresh your memory, Dr. Shoemaker had diagnosed Rick with toxic encephalopathy, an autoimmune illness resulting from prolonged exposure to toxins, in 2005. Symptoms often include memory loss, personality changes, increased irritability, insidious onset of concentration difficulties, involuntary movements (Parkinsonism), fatigue, seizures, arm strength problems, and depression. Toxic encephalopathy had a confirmed DSM code for use by health professionals for listing a patient's diagnosis for insurance purposes, and it was in alignment with Rick's symptoms. With Bredesen's team investigating the factors associated with Alzheimer's disease, their research for Type 3 confirmed toxic origins and noted symptoms to those of toxic encephalopathy.

In further review of related research, in the bio-medical journal, *Aging*, I discovered this article by Dr. Bredesen: "Inhalational Alzheimer's Disease: an Unrecognized—and Treatable—Epidemic." It appeared just two months prior to Rick's death. Indeed, this neurological inflammatory illness has long gone unrecognized, but now science has revealed that it is treatable! How I wish I had been able to share this fantastic news with Rick! He had suffered throughout the duration of his illness without the toxic nature of his illness ever being truly legitimized.

There it was—more validation of Dr. Shoemaker's brilliant work, receiving kudos from Dr. Bredesen. Both scientists have tirelessly revealed research so revolutionary in supporting both the prevention and healing from the scourge of neurological debilitation. As Dr. Bredesen wrote:

> "Over the past two decades, elegant work from Dr. R. Shoemaker and his colleagues has demonstrated unequivocally that biotoxins such as mycotoxins are associated with a broad range of symptoms, including cognitive decline ... These researchers and clinicians identified a constellation of symptoms, signs, genetic predisposition (HLA-DR/DQ haplotypes), and laboratory abnormalities characteristic of patients exposed to, and sensitive to, these biotoxins. The resulting syndrome has been designated chronic inflammatory response syndrome (CIRS)."[4]

In summary, nine years after Rick's diagnosis of toxic encephalopathy, a neurologist diagnosed him with Lewy body dementia. Environmental factors and toxic exposures are suspect as *dementogens*, a term used to describe toxic agents that may lead to cognitive decline.

Both toxic encephalopathy and LBD accurately defined the manifestations of Rick's symptoms and behavior, as would Type 3 (toxic-related) Alzheimer's. The common denominator was brain inflammation created by a combination of underlying issues—toxicity, genetics, stress, infections, and other contributing causes, facts that are now scientifically validated.

Bredesen's team designed a protocol to address the mechanisms that drive the process of cognitive decline in Alzheimer's disease. The protocol, including detoxification among other therapies, helped patients to awaken from the fog of cognitive decline. The few LBD patients who were part of his research study shared some of the same mechanisms for neurodegeneration associated with Type 3 (toxin-related) Alzheimer's disease and were more challenged in their recovery.

As research continues into brain diseases and these biochemical mechanisms become better understood, a new paradigm is now recognized for both preventing and recovering from brain inflammation. Dr. Bredesen's research team continues to document increasing numbers of patients who are reawakening from Alzheimer's and helping to prevent others from navigating their own neurological nightmares. As he wrote:

> "Type 3 Alzheimer's disease is the result of exposure to specific toxins, and is most commonly inhalational (IAD), a phenotypic manifestation of chronic inflammatory response syndrome (CIRS), due to biotoxins such as mycotoxins. The appropriate recognition of IAD as a potentially important pathogenetic condition in patients with cognitive decline offers the opportunity for successful treatment of a large number of patients whose current prognoses, in the absence of accurate diagnosis, are grave."[5]

This new information about a toxic type of Alzheimer's brought up a question. Was Rick's neurological condition properly diagnosed as LBD or Type 3 AD? At the time of his death, the toxic connections to Alzheimer's were in the well-documented research of Bredesen's team, but not yet widespread in mainstream.

Fortunately, one of the few people who could offer such insights was Dr. Bredesen himself. I graciously received this reply to my inquiry:

> "Professor John Trojanowski, a well-known neuropathologist from the University of Pennsylvania, found that about 70% of patients with AD not only have amyloid plaques and tau tangles, but also have Lewy bodies and TDP-43 (TDP-43 is characteristic of frontotemporal dementia and ALS). So, there is some overlap between these syndromes.
>
> In your husband's case, he likely had Lewy bodies as well as amyloid and tau, so very possibly some degree of LBD and type 3 AD. If his symptoms corresponded more to those I listed in type 3, then the main issue was probably type 3 AD; whereas, if he had symptoms typical of LBD, such as visual hallucinations, then the dominant pathology was probably LBD (and if he had a PET scan, that could also distinguish).

However, as you noted, doctors tend to focus on pathological diagnoses instead of root causes, and in either case, the root cause is likely toxins, whether from inorganics, organics, or biotoxins (and his lab values support biotoxins as a key player)."

At long last, a leading researcher of the characteristics and causes of dementias provided answers regarding Rick's illness. Rick aligned with the symptoms of both LBD and Type 3 (toxic) Alzheimer's. As research has confirmed, dementia patients can have both the amyloid plaques and tau tangles associated with Alzheimer's as well as Lewy bodies and TDP-43, characteristic of frontotemporal dementia. Included in the report of Rick's final neuropsychological evaluation stating that his performance is consistent with a neurodegenerative disorder, such as a subcortical dementia with frontotemporal dementia as a possibility. This further legitimized the organic nature of his illness.

Had all of Rick's tests from functional practitioners confirming the toxic roots of his illness been accepted by his conventional treatment team years earlier, undoubtedly our journey would have been decidedly different. By sharing details of our journey, you will find many of the revelations from it contained in the chapters that follow.

(See chapter 19 for more details about this revolutionary evaluation and treatment program; and Appendix F).

A Legacy Offering More than Hope

While Rick's journey is over, legions of others are currently seeking answers to the erratic nature of their own debilitating health issues. We are being bombarded by toxins from our environment, stressed out from our hectic lifestyles, and devour increasingly nutritionally bankrupt foods in the standard American diet (SAD). Sad indeed when these factors, combined with others highlighted in this book, are igniting firestorms within bodies of all ages. We are all vulnerable. This is a wake-up call for us all!

Now, we can cling to more than hope during these inflammatory times. With growing awareness of these root realities, we have the power to influence and modify our own health destinies. By partnering with practitioners who recognize these inflammatory agents, coupled with their healing arsenals of lifestyle interventions, precise evaluations and transformative therapies, a promising future can be reclaimed.

Really, what we're finding out is toxic mold exposure is a pandemic issue. It's affecting everybody in their homes, schools, cars, and workplace. And to be able to identify those symptoms early, before they take you down, and if you've already been taken down, then what are you going to do with all the things that you've learned along the way?[6]

Margaret Christensen, MD

The remainder of this book describes the interconnections of chronic inflammatory illnesses and how evolving science is leading to greater possibilities for vibrant wellness. It also highlights ways to reduce your own risks of inflammation in today's toxic times.

Additionally, with care issues a priority to all on a similar journey, these are also highlighted, required in navigating this terrain. I have also included some strategies that proved essential as my lifeline for sustaining my spirit through the turbulence of uncharted waters.

Part 2

Living in
Inflammatory Times

Chapter 13
Bodies on Fire

Addressing metal and chemical toxins and all their downstream effects on
our biology is essential if we are to address our chronic disease epidemic and
the burden of mood, memory, attention, and behavior disorders.[1]

Mark Hyman, MD

The Roots of Chronic Inflammation

Rick's body and brain were on fire, but doctors were not tracking inflammation, nor the underlying reasons that had ignited it. That is what made Rick's journey so frustrating, and now so compelling for me to share. This section highlights the critical need for recognizing and addressing the root causes of inflammation so that the long battle Rick and others have experienced might be avoided.

The phrase "canary in the coal mine" references an earlier practice in which birds were sent into coal mines to see if they survived the toxic fumes before it was considered safe for coalminers to enter. Rick was one among millions of "canaries," living in an increasingly toxic world that helped trigger the inflammation that brought him down.

It was not until after Rick's death that I was fully able to assemble the collection of information and insights as to why his health mysteriously collapsed. Toxicity from chemicals, biotoxins, and heavy metals were not the only inflammatory factors at play. His case serves as a 21st century model of what the human body is now experiencing and why this is a matter of concern to all of us.

His chronic digestive issues were screaming for attention, but his conventional treatment team did not yet recognize the interrelationships of the gut-brain connection (see chapter 16). Prior to the onset of his debilitating neurological issues, Rick was being treated for periodontal disease; bacterial infections are linked to brain issues. His preferred diet of refined carbohydrates and refined sugars, which are inflammatory by nature, also lacked vital nutrients. These contributing factors were never explored or linked to the manifestation of his illness. Now with inflammation recognized as an underlying cause of most diseases, it's important to know more about what ignites it.

The Rise of Mysterious Maladies

During the 1980s, Rick Irvin, then a toxicologist at Texas A&M University, envisioned the dangerous impact chemicals would have on health: "Chemicals have replaced bacteria and viruses as the main threat to human health ... The diseases we're beginning to see as the major cause of death in the latter part of this century and into the 21ˢᵗ century are diseases of chemical origin."[2]

Long before toxicity had impacted our own lives, Rick and I watched *A Civil Action*, a movie starring John Travolta. First released in book form, it is based on the true story of a leather factory in Woburn, Massachusetts, and the chemical trichloroethylene, an industrial solvent used in the tanning process. When residents started developing cancers and toxin-related health problems at an abnormally high rate, they filed a class action lawsuit against the factory and won.

Coincidentally, during that same time, Rick's father had owned a leather tanning factory just 30 miles away from Woburn in Peabody, Massachusetts. For decades, his family had lived in a house just yards from the factory. While growing up, Rick remembered a favorite childhood memory: jumping regularly on a tall stack of tanned hides for fun. No one recognized any danger from the chemicals used in their processing—formaldehyde, xylene, naphthalene, and tannic and phosphoric acids, among others. When the factory closed in the 1990s, the Environmental Protection Agency (EPA) mandated a massive cleanup of the chemicals before the land could be developed for residential use.

Rick spent 30 years as a vocational rehabilitation consultant, hired by attorneys as an expert witness in personal injury cases, representing clients who become disabled or died from known or suspected worksite environmental problems. He even testified in a class action suit filed—ironically—by EPA employees who were suffering from Sick Building Syndrome (SBS), where building occupants experience health effects related to time spent in a building with toxic agents.

Many of the clients in these cases presented with seemingly unrelated symptoms: tingling and muscle weakness; persistent cough; burning, itchy eyes; joint pain; prolonged fatigue; headaches; GI issues; and depression and anxiety. These maladies were not always from working in a chemical plant. Sometimes, it was a result of mold from water-damaged buildings, long-term exposure to the off-gassing of chemicals like benzene, ammonia, toluene, and formaldehyde in office furnishings and newly installed carpet, the release of volatile organic compounds (VOCs) in paint, and others.

The doctors treating these patients diagnosed a litany of different autoimmune diseases—Guillain-Barre syndrome, lupus, rheumatoid arthritis, chronic fatigue syndrome, fibromyalgia, multiple sclerosis, irritable bowel syndrome (IBS), among others.

The question I asked long before Rick got sick: "How can these workplace exposures cause one employee to become too sick and exhausted to work, while the coworker at the next desk remains healthy?" Enter the genetics. As Dr. Shoemaker revealed in Rick's case, some people are born with a genotype that makes them poor detoxifiers.

Today's Ticking Time Bombs

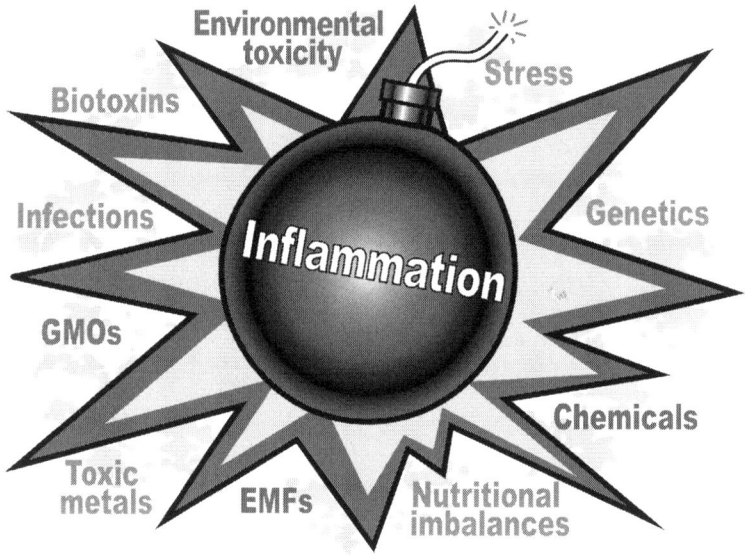

There are two things most physicians never learn in medical school:
1) The role of nutrition and food in health and disease; and
2) The role of toxins and the importance of detoxification in health and
disease. And they are probably the two most important things we need to
know to cure disease and create health.[3]

Mark Hyman, MD

Twenty-first century risk factors have turned us into ticking time bombs. The food we eat, the air we breathe, the water we drink, the medications we take, manufacturing and agricultural practices, and the electronic revolution—all have roles contributing to the epidemic of chronic inflammatory illnesses:

- You may wonder why you're gaining weight, even though you exercise and watch what you eat. When the body is unable to adequately process toxins, it enrobes them in fat cells and stores them in your tissues, often as visceral belly fat surrounding your organs.

- Digestive issues usually arise, too. The vital connection between the gut's microbiome and overall immune health is now well-documented. When the gut isn't working right, your immune system can go haywire, causing your body's infection-fighting cytokines to overproduce and attack your tissues and cells. This causes more inflammation and autoimmunity.

- Your hormones run amok. Your brain gets foggy, confused, or worse, and you're very likely to experience varying degrees of depression, anxiety, or other mood changes.

- Statistics demonstrate we are experiencing more cancers, dementias, obesity, diabetes, and more alphabet maladies like ADHD, ADD, OCD, ALS, MS, AD, PD, and other neurological issues. During the last few decades, we've been relentlessly bombarded by environmental assaults from electromagnetic frequencies (EMFs) and genetically modified organisms (GMOs).

Toxins are now the primary cause of chronic disease. They are driving much of what we see as clinicians. We need to reckon with the fact that our population is incredibly sick, and toxins are a major driver.[4]

Joseph Pizzorno, ND

Chapter 14
Root Cause Realities

The term, *root cause(s)*, refers to the underlying agents of chronic inflammation, e.g., toxic heavy metals, chemicals, environmental toxins, nutritional deficiencies, sedentary lifestyles, sleep issues, hormone imbalances, chronic infections, stress, and others. These hidden triggers can lead to chronic health conditions unless they are identified and properly treated.

Unprecedented Toxic Exposures

Toxins are poisons. We live in a world where it's impossible to escape from toxic exposure—it's not a matter of if you're toxic, but to what degree. Toxic exposure is cumulative, beginning in the womb and compounded throughout our lives. A few examples:

- Research commissioned in 2004 by the Environmental Working Group (EWG), entitled "Body Burden—The Pollution in Newborns," revealed that the umbilical cord blood in newborns contained an average of 200 industrial chemicals and a total of 287 chemicals, with 180 known to cause cancer in humans or animals. Of those, 217 are toxic to the brain and nervous system, and 208 cause birth defects or abnormal development in animal tests.[1]

- The breast milk from Inuit mothers in the remote Artic wilderness is so contaminated with PCBs that the FDA would classify it as hazardous waste if evaluated for human consumption.[2]

- 60% of US women carry loads of PCB187 sufficient to double their risk of breast cancer.[3]

- 33% of Americans have lead levels high enough to double the risk of Amyotrophic Lateral Sclerosis (ALS).[4]

- 25% are exposed to enough aluminum to double Alzheimer's risk.[5]

- 25% carry enough PCBs to *double* the odds of rheumatoid arthritis.[6]

These statistics are alarming and serve as a wake-up call for all of us and our healthcare providers to recognize toxic impact. We are now inhaling, ingesting, and absorbing toxins at record rates. Even small, daily doses of toxins become cumulative over time, especially in those who are genetically unable to properly detoxify.

We typically think of toxins originating from the foods we eat, the water we drink, or the air we breathe. But toxins are present in the lotions and potions we lather on our bodies; the flame retardant mattresses laced with

PBDE; the expansive list of cleaning products and detergents; fragrances in colognes, candles, air fresheners, and dryer sheets; and the plethora of plastics containing bisphenol A (BPA). They are invisible as in our wireless networks, emitting radiation potentially damaging to our DNA.

We've acquired ravenous appetites for nutritionally deficient, processed, and "fake" foods manufactured with sugars, refined flours, artificial sweeteners, flavors, colors, salts, and more chemicals. Even our once-pure whole foods are laced with more pesticides, herbicides, hormones, antibiotics, and fungicides, and are increasingly genetically modified.

Toxins of any kind ultimately poison the mitochondria, the energy power-house of our cells, causing a myriad of problems. According to Dr. Joseph Pizzorno, toxins can:

- Poison the enzymes needed to manufacture molecules, cells and produce energy. This inhibits the production of hemoglobin in the blood and lowers the body's capacity to prevent free radical damage, which accelerates aging.

- Damage organs and systems if your digestive tract, liver, and kidneys are unable to detox effectively.

- Displace structural minerals, resulting in weaker bones.

- Damage DNA, increasing the rate of aging and degeneration.

- Interfere with hormones and cause imbalances, e.g., arsenic disrupts thyroid hormone receptors on the cells so cells cannot properly communicate with thyroid hormones.

- Modify genetic expression. Toxins can activate or suppress our genes in undesirable ways. This is a major reason why certain health issues span generations.

- Damage cell membranes, e.g., insulin is unable to signal the cells to absorb more sugar.[7]

Chemicals

> *Unfortunately, our bodies were never designed to protect themselves against this chemical onslaught. As a result, our systems usually fail to process and remove most of these chemicals once they have entered our bodies, so their levels start building up inside us. Consequently, every single human on the face of this earth is now permanently contaminated with these modern synthetic chemicals.[8]*
>
> Dr. Paula Baillie-Hamilton

It's estimated that every second 683 pounds (310 kilograms) of toxic chemicals are released into our air, land, and water by industrial facilities around the world. This constitutes more than 21 billion pounds of toxic chemicals released into our global environment annually.[9]

According to the EPA Inventory Update Reporting program, an estimated 27 trillion pounds of chemicals were produced in or imported into the United States per year in the last decade, which is the equivalent of approximately 74 billion pounds/day (nearly 250 pounds per person). This figure does not include fuels, pesticides, pharmaceuticals, or food products. It is also estimated that the use of chemicals will double by 2024.[10] The 2019 report issued by the Centers for Disease Control and Prevention (CDC) states that an average of 108 toxic chemicals are now found in *every* U.S. resident.[11]

The National Resources Defense Council, an environmental action group, reports that of the 80,000 known environmental chemicals, only 200 have been tested by the EPA. According to the Environmental Working Group, cosmetics and personal care products contribute to more chemical exposure than almost any other consumer products and have less government oversight.

American women use an average of twelve personal care products daily that contain 168 different chemicals. Men use an average of six personal care products daily, containing 85 different chemicals. The chemicals in these items can enter the body through the skin, inhalation, and ingestion, and pose the same risks as food chemicals.[12] Since 2009, a total of 595 cosmetic manufacturers have reported using nearly 90 chemicals more than 73,000 products, many linked to cancer, birth defects, and reproductive issues.[13] They include:

- Phthalates, parabens, and other toxic ingredients frequently formulated in hair products, lotions, and fragrances

- Aluminum in deodorants

- Low volatile organic compounds (VOC) in paints and paint thinners

- Fluoride and triclosan in toothpaste

- Teflon in cookware

- Oxybenzone is one of the most used sunscreen active ingredients, found in more than 60% of non-mineral sunscreens. This and other chemicals included in some sunscreens have insufficient data and data gaps for safety.[14]

- Lead in lipsticks

- Formaldehyde, toluene, and DBP (Dibutyl phthalate), the "toxic trio" in nail polish

- Triclosan was banned for use in over-the-counter antibacterial soaps and body washes in 2016, but still approved for use in toothpaste, mouthwash and shaving cream, as reported by the FDA.[15] It was banned for use in hand sanitizers in 2019.[16]

Research has identified nearly a dozen known industrial neurotoxicants, including lead, methylmercury, polychlorinated biphenyls, arsenic, toluene, and fluoride that are harmful to brain development in human fetuses and infants.[17] Continuing research suggests that even minute traces of many common chemicals—touted by industry and some scientists to be biologically safe—can affect cells and proper functioning of the endocrine system.

As Donna Jackson Nakazawa describes in her book, *The Autoimmune Epidemic:* "When our endocrine system's exquisite communication network goes on the blink, the immune system's network can go haywire as well." Take for example, the rather ubiquitous toxin, bisphenol A (BPA), now confirmed as an "endocrine disruptor" and until recently used in a multitude of plastic products. Small doses over time disrupt normal endocrine function and natural hormonal signals, which affects the immune system and the body's resistance to disease. "Researchers now understand that a wide array of environmental chemicals can act as endocrine disruptors, affecting us at much lower doses than scientists previously thought possible," says Nakazawa.[18]

Heavy Metals

Mercury, lead, arsenic, cadmium, and aluminum are among the heavy metals linked to neurological issues, cancer, and organ damage. They naturally occur in water and soil and can contaminate food sources such as fish and fresh produce at levels considered unsafe. *Consumer Reports*, the publication of a non-profit consumer protection organization, found heavy metals in all 50 packaged baby food items they tested for lead, cadmium, or inorganic arsenic.[19]

Mercury is widely used in the mining and manufacturing of many consumer products and the resulting industrial waste has polluted our waterways. Traces of mercury are now found in most fish and shellfish, some with higher levels than the Food and Drug Administration (FDA) and the Environmental Protection Agency (EPA) advise. Especially at risk are pregnant women or those who may become pregnant, nursing mothers, and young children.

Mercury has been used in vaccines and dental amalgams. An extensive epidemiological study conducted by the National Institutes for Health (NIH), revealed a high correlation between dental fillings and chronic diseases, including autoimmune, neurological and mood disorders, cancer and immune dysfunction, cardiovascular issues, hormonal imbalances, reproductive problems, and oral health problems, including periodontal disease.[20] Mercury is also contained in fluorescent and energy-efficient compact fluorescent (CFL) light bulbs that come with warning labels instructing consumers to dispose of broken bulbs as hazardous waste.

Even low levels of lead can impair brain development in fetuses, infants and young children and are linked to ongoing health issues including anemia, hearing impairment, cardiovascular disease, neurological issues, and behavioral problems.[21]

Biotoxins

Naturally occurring toxins, such as mold, certain dinoflagellates, algae, and Lyme bacterial complex, are classified as biotoxins. These microbes can produce poisons that make us sick. (See also Appendix B: The Ticking Time Bomb of Lyme.) Chronic Inflammatory Response Syndrome (CIRS) is a condition affecting those who are genetically compromised to effectively detoxify biotoxins. Biotoxic exposure can result in serious health issues affecting the neuroimmune, gastrointestinal, vascular, and endocrine systems.[22]

Mycotoxicosis is a disease resulting from exposure to a mycotoxin, compounds that are naturally produced by certain types of molds. As noted in the 2018 research study, "Effects of mycotoxins on neuropsychiatric symptoms and immune processes," People exposed to molds and mycotoxins present with symptoms affecting multiple organs, including the lungs, musculoskeletal system, as well as the central and peripheral nervous systems ... These toxins can cause multisystemic effects, including gastrointestinal, cardiovascular, and neuropsychiatric complications."[23]

Dementogens made by molds such as *Stachybotrys, Aspergillus, Penicillium* and others were found repeatedly in Type 3 Alzheimer's patients. Research links mold to an estimated 500,000 Alzheimer's cases in the US alone, so it important to have a mycotoxin test, especially if you or loved ones have noticed cognitive decline.[24]

Sixty to sixty-five percent clinically of Alzheimer's patients, the type of Alzheimer's they have is largely inhalation[al] Alzheimer's. It's what they're breathing that has triggered the inflammation eventually causing all the scar, the crud in the brain that progresses into Alzheimer's.[25]

Dr. Tom O'Bryan

Water Pollution

More than 300 pollutants contaminate US water supplies, with more than half of them found in tap water. According to the EWG's analysis of almost 20 million public records, these pollutants are not subject to health or safety limits and can legally be present in any amount.[26] Studies of municipal water supplies have revealed unsafe levels of heavy metals, hormones, pharmaceuticals such as birth control pills and antidepressants, pesticides, fecal matter, toxic chemicals, and even jet fuel.

In 2014, dangerously high lead levels in Flint, Michigan's water made headlines nationwide. Residents complained of discolored foul-tasting water that was making people sick. Flint officials had failed to treat the water contaminated from the lead that was leaching out from aging pipes into thousands of homes. A 2015 study confirmed that blood-lead levels in children in Flint had doubled or nearly tripled from the previous year.

The problem was further compounded with the discovery of fecal coliform bacteria in Flint water, linked to the city's failure to maintain sufficient levels of disinfecting chlorine. More health issues arose when Flint's corrective measure—adding more chlorine to its water without addressing other underlying issues—created elevated levels of total trihalomethanes (TTHM), cancer-causing chemicals that are a by-product of water chlorination.[27]

Nearly three-quarters of Americans now drink fluoridated water.[28] Fluoride, a known neurotoxin, has been added to municipal water supplies for 70 years, in the belief that it reduces tooth decay. However, decades of research demonstrates that while the topical application of fluoride has such benefits, drinking fluoridated water is largely ineffective for this purpose.

An accumulating body of research has raised numerous red flags about the potential harm for even low levels of fluoride. A report issued by the U.S. National Research Council (NRC) expressed concern about fluoride's link to dementia: "Studies of populations exposed to different concentrations of fluoride should be undertaken to evaluate neurochemical changes that may be associated with dementia. Consideration should be given to assessing effects from chronic exposure, effects that might be delayed or occur late-in-life, and individual susceptibility."[29]

In a joint study identifying developmental neurotoxicants conducted by the Harvard School of Public Health and Icahn School of Medicine at Mount Sinai, the senior author of the study, Phillipe Grandjean, stated: "Fluoride seems to fit in with lead, mercury, and other poisons that cause chemical brain drain ... The effect of each toxicant may seem small, but the combined damage on a population scale can be serious, especially because the brain power of the next generation is crucial to all of us."[30]

In November 2016, several environmental groups filed a petition calling on the EPA to ban the deliberate addition of fluoridating chemicals to the drinking water under provisions in the Toxic Substances Control Act (TSCA). The petition included more than 2,500 pages of scientific documentation that detailed the risks of water fluoridation to human health.

In 2017, with the denial of that petition, the members of the environmental coalition filed a complaint against EPA. "We believe this lawsuit is an unprecedented opportunity to end the practice once and for all in the U.S., and potentially throughout the world, based on the well-documented neurotoxicity of fluoride," stated Michael Connett, Fluoride Action Network's attorney and advisor.[31]

The trial was finally held in June 2020 and the judge had yet to make his ruling as of January 2021.[32]

Electromagnetic Fields (EMFs)

Putting in tens of millions of 5G antennae without a single biological test of safety has got to be about the stupidest idea anyone has had in the history of the world.[33]

Dr. Martin L. Pall

These are emitted from man-made sources—electric currents and voltages from the power system. You are exposed to these invisible sources of radiation from your computer, Wi-Fi router, Bluetooth cell phone, TV, microwaves and other appliances, MRIs, power lines, and smart meters.

Laboratory studies have pointed to EMFs affecting biological processes on a cellular level, such as changes in human nerve function. However, despite accumulating experimental evidence, the underlying mechanisms are poorly understood.[34] Mounting evidence demonstrates the technology is not without risk.

Research conducted by the World Health Organization (WHO)/International Agency for Research on Cancer (IARC) classified radiofrequency electromagnetic fields as possibly carcinogenic to humans, based on an increased risk for brain cancer.[35] The National Toxicology Program conducted a 10-year study to assess long-term health effects from high levels of radio frequency (RFR) from 2G and 3G cellphones in rats and mice. It provided clear evidence of tumors in the hearts of male rats, and some evidence of tumors in the brains and adrenal glands.[36] A review of several studies on low-frequency EMFs point to the potential risks these energy fields may cause, including neurological and psychiatric problems. Some scientists also attribute this technology to a potential risk for wide range of symptoms, but more research is needed to determine the effects upon human health.[37]

As Theresa Dale, PhD, CCN, NP writes, EMFs can act like antennas, sending and receiving information magnified by the toxic metals inside our bodies:

> "Heavy metals can weaken our field through their frequency outputs by modulating compatible frequency components of the body resulting in a weakening of the field, thereby causing unhealthy biochemical changes. If you have accumulated toxic metals in your brain, and since your brain is an antenna, you can actually receive more cell phone radiation, which in turn can cause the microbes in your system to overreact and create more potent mycotoxins.
>
> This can create a never-ending vicious cycle between the microbes and metals in your body and your exposure to electromagnetic fields, which can lead to hypersensitivity. I have seen that a high percentage of illness including chronic infections are caused, and/or aggravated, by electromagnetic field exposure. Then chronic fatigue, fibromyalgia and other chronic pain syndromes can easily develop or worsen."[38]

Experts tracking these connections are sounding the alarm about the 5G networks increasing across the American landscape:

> *Wireless radiation has biological effects. Period. This is no longer a subject for debate when you look at PubMed and the peer-reviewed literature. These effects are seen in all life forms: plants, animals, insects, microbes. In humans, we have clear evidence of cancer now: there is no question. We have evidence of DNA damage, cardiomyopathy, which is the precursor of congestive heart failure, neuropsychiatric effects …*
>
> *5G is an untested application of a technology that we know is harmful; we know it from the science. In academics, this is called human subjects' research.*[39]
>
> Sharon Goldberg, MD

From his decades of researching an ocean of epidemiology and toxicology, Dr. Pizzorno sounds the alarm awakening us to the realities of toxicity upon our health: "We are doomed to huge burdens of disease if we don't get our act together on this," he says, emphasizing that "the medical community needs to take the toxin issue seriously, recognizing it as the dire public health issue that it is."[40]

Other Root Cause Realities

While toxins are wreaking havoc on our health, they are not solely responsible for the epidemic of chronic inflammation. Nutritional deficiencies, stress, genetic susceptibility, chronic infections, and hormonal imbalances also weaken the body's defenses and cause a cascade of symptoms.

Stress

> *Stress is a factor in most cases of cognitive decline, but an especially strong one in type 3 (toxic) Alzheimer's disease.*[41]
>
> Dale Bredesen, MD

Daily life is filled with countless moments that aggravate or rattle us—traffic jams, watching or listening to news reports, or standing in long lines. Even scanning social media posts can fire up the stress response.

Ironically, I'm writing this during the 2020-21 coronavirus pandemic, which generated global stress all around the planet. People are consumed with fear on multiple fronts—of contracting the virus, the economic impact of business closings, unemployment, the scarcity of resources, and other collateral damage.

Chronic stress ravages the immune system, activating cortisol, "the stress hormone" in response. Cortisol suppresses the immune system by switching off inflammatory responses that protect against infection, making us more vulnerable to viral infections and diseases. It also suppresses levels of serotonin and dopamine—the "happy hormones" that help regulate mood—leading to anxiety, depression, irritability, low self-esteem, mood swings, and more.[42] Chronic stress can also activate a cascade of potentially damaging effects to our organs, muscles, and metabolic processes. High levels of cortisol are linked to weight gain, cardiovascular and brain issues, headaches, asthma, insomnia, skin problems, and others.[43]

Dr. Bredesen's research team has shown that the onset of cognitive decline, particularly in patients with toxic exposures, usually coincides with a time of great stress.

Changes in Our Food, Changes in Our Health

> *We now have the most addictive and chemical-laden food in the history of humanity.*[44]
>
> Ocean Robbins, Food Revolution Network

Our food-crop soils have become anemic, stripped of the ninety or so nutrients essential to human health from fertilizers, pesticides, herbicides, irrigation, acid rain, and other related factors. Nutrient deficiencies that result in the human body depress and kill cells in the immune system rendering the body more vulnerable to illness and disease.[45]

Randall Fitzgerald

The death of soils at the hands of agriculture is manifesting as deadly diseases in our bodies. Rising concentrations of toxic farm chemicals and declining nutrient levels in our foods have been revealed as root causes of cancer, heart disease, diabetes and even obesity. This killer isn't just a killer. It's a serial killer.[46]

From online video event at Eat4Earth.org

Whole, living foods grown in nutrient-rich soils contain most of the elements needed for our bodies to function properly. However, American soil, once brimming with minerals needed for healthy bodies, has lost much of its fertility. Due to changes in agricultural practices over the last century, our once mineral-packed soil has been stripped of its nutrients.

The degradation of soil microorganisms needed for plant health is also having a detrimental effect on our own internal microbiome. In 2004, researchers from the University of Texas published a landmark study of U.S. Department of Agriculture nutritional data. They discovered "reliable declines" in the amount of protein, calcium, phosphorus, iron, riboflavin (vitamin B_2), and vitamin C in 43 different vegetables and fruits over the past half century.[47] This loss of vital nutrients causes nutritional deficiencies that depress and kill cells in the immune system, rendering the body more vulnerable to illness and disease.

In addition, many conventionally grown fresh fruits and vegetables are laced with poisonous pesticides. The EWG's *2021 Shopper's Guide to Pesticides in Produce* includes data demonstrating that nearly 70% of conventionally grown produce in the U.S. is contaminated with pesticide residues.[48]

Strawberries topped the list, with a single sample of strawberries showing 20 different pesticides. Before testing, all produce was washed and peeled, demonstrating that washing alone does not remove all pesticide residues. USDA testing found 225 different pesticides on popular produce items Americans consume daily.[49]

EWG's 2021 "Dirty Dozen" (an annual ranking) of fruits and vegetables with the most pesticide residues ranked conventionally grown spinach in second place, with kale, collards, and mustard greens tied for third.

Recognized as a rich source of vitamins and antioxidants, kale's popularity has skyrocketed over the past few years. Unfortunately, the levels and types of pesticide residues detected on kale, collards, and mustard greens have also increased—20 different pesticides were detected in a single sample. According to the 2017 USDA data reported by EWG, nearly 60% of kale samples sold in the U.S. were contaminated with residues of a pesticide the EPA considers a possible human carcinogen.[50]

On a positive note, EWG also publishes their annual "Clean Fifteen" listing featuring the cleanest of conventionally grown fruits and vegetables. Nearly 70% of these produce samples had no pesticide residues.

As the author of *Fancy Fruits and Extraordinary Vegetables* (no longer available) and the former vice president of consumer affairs for a national fresh produce association, my primary responsibility was promoting healthy eating and health-enhancing lifestyles. As science continues to reveal the health consequences from agrichemicals used in food production, selecting organic produce and fruits and vegetables from the Clean Fifteen list, as well as other organic foods, is now vital to reduce toxic exposures.

Genetically Modified Organisms (GMOs)

Dramatic increases in genetically modified foods (GMOs) have infiltrated the American food system, with questionable evidence as to their safety. Genetically modifying food includes the artificial insertion of genes from bacteria, viruses, insects, animals, or even humans into the DNA of food crops or animals. It is estimated that upwards of 75% of processed foods found in our supermarkets—from soda to soup, crackers to condiments—contain genetically engineered ingredients.[51]

Many processed foods contain genetically engineered ingredients in vegetable oils, corn syrups and sweeteners. Currently, at least 90% of corn (corn syrup is a widely used sweetener; cornstarch is used in soups and sauces) soy, canola, and cottonseed oils sold in the United States are genetically engineered.[52] For a comprehensive list, consult the Institute for Responsible Technology's website.

Despite findings by the FDA that GMOs could pose serious risks to health, labeling for GMO foods has not been required.[53] As a result, consumers have no way to determine whether GMOs are in the foods they are buying. That's about to change. In 2018, USDA's Agricultural Marketing Service's (AMS) highly anticipated "GMO" labeling rule morphed into a "bioengineered" labeling rule, which has been finalized.

The National Bioengineered Food Disclosure Law directed USDA to establish a national mandatory standard for disclosing foods that are or may be bioengineered. The standard defines bioengineered foods as those that contain detectable genetic material that has been modified through certain lab techniques and cannot be created through conventional breeding or found in nature. The mandatory compliance date is January 1, 2022.[54] Unfortunately, the final rule for this National Bioengineered Food Disclosure Standard fails to provide an accurate and transparent message about which foods contain genetic engineering or genetically modified organisms (GMOs).[55]

Studies have demonstrated that genetically modified foods can leave residues in the body, with the potential for creating long-term problems. Animal studies on GMOs have shown organ damage, gastrointestinal and immune system disorders, accelerated aging and infertility. The American Academy of Environmental Medicine encourages doctors to prescribe non-GMO diets for their patients.[56]

According to the 2014 study, "Genetically Engineered Crops, Glyphosate and the Deterioration of Health in the United States of America," the combination of GMOs and the accelerated use of glyphosate is linked to the dramatic rate of chronic disease, with an estimated 25% of the US population suffering from multiple chronic diseases.[57]

The rate of chronic health conditions among children in the United States increased from 12.8% in 1994 to 26.6% in 2006, particularly for asthma, obesity, and behavior and learning problems. During the same time period, "there has been an exponential increase in the amount of glyphosate applied to food crops and in the percentage of GMO food crops planted." These findings suggest environmental triggers rather than genetic or age-related causes.[58]

A 2013 paper published in the scientific journal, *Entropy*, explains the connection between glyphosate and gastrointestinal disorders, obesity, diabetes, heart disease, depression, autism, infertility, cancer, and Alzheimer's disease. According to the authors: "Glyphosate enhances the damaging effects of other food borne chemical residues and environmental toxins. Negative impact on the body is insidious and manifests slowly over time as inflammation damages cellular systems throughout the body."[59]

Over the decades, the production of meat, dairy, poultry, and seafood has also changed. Antibiotics and hormones have proven benefits for increasing production in meat and dairy products, but their use is not without controversy because of the impact on human health. Larger edible species of fish like tuna, shark, tilefish, and swordfish carry a heavy toxic load from the mercury in their flesh, while those who eat farm-raised fish risk contamination from the bacteria and antibiotics used in the farming process.

Only a few decades ago, our bodies were naturally fueled with vital nutrients from whole foods, grown without pesticides or the infusion of antibiotics, hormones, and other agents. The standard American diet has been dramatically transformed as we rely more and more on the convenience of processed foods to sustain our fast-paced culture. Processed foods are notoriously high in added sugars, harmful fats, artificial ingredients, and chemicals—a lot of empty calories with little nutritional value.

Gluten Sensitivities

Gluten is what I call a "silent germ."
It can inflict lasting damage without your knowing it.[60]
David Perlmutter, MD

With the predominance of GMO wheat in our food system, gluten sensitivity has risen dramatically in the past few decades. Gluten is also found in other grains and considered as one of the most common food additives used in processed foods and personal care items.

As reported in *Grain Brain—The Surprising Truth about Wheat, Carbs and Sugar—Your Brain's Silent Killers* by David Perlmutter, MD., the *Lancet* featured a well-respected researcher in gluten sensitivity and the brain, Professor Marios Hadjivassilious. He stated: "Our data suggest that gluten sensitivity is common in patients with neurological disease of unknown cause and may have etiological significance." It often serves as a silent inflammatory agent since "an estimated 99% of people whose immune systems react negatively to gluten don't even know it. Hadjivassilious continues, "Gluten sensitivity can be primarily, and at times, exclusively, a neurological disease."[61] This means people with gluten sensitivity can have brain function issues without even having GI issues!

Gluten sensitivity is caused by elevated levels of antibodies which can turn on specific genes. Once activated, inflammatory cytokines are highly antagonist to the brain, damaging tissue and making the brain vulnerable to dysfunction and disease.

Artificial Sweeteners

Artificial sweeteners, heralded by some as the darlings of the food industry for their no-calorie sweetening power in soft drinks, fruit-flavored drinks, cereals, frozen desserts, and foods labeled as "zero," "light" or "low calorie," have been embraced by many calorie-counting and diabetic consumers. Artificial sweeteners are also found in pharmaceuticals. However, numerous studies have revealed these sweeteners' toxic truth.

Aspartame has been linked to Alzheimer's disease and other dementias, autoimmune and metabolic disorders, cancers and more.[62] Additional studies have shown its connection to other behavioral and cognitive issues including learning problems, headaches, seizures, migraines, irritable moods, anxiety, depression, and insomnia.[63]

It contains three primary chemicals and, upon digestion, breaks down into three components (aspartic acid, phenylalanine, and methanol). Aspartic acid is in a class of chemicals known as excitotoxins. "Abnormally high levels of excitotoxins have been shown in hundreds of animals studies to cause damage to areas of the brain unprotected by the blood-brain barrier and a variety of chronic diseases arising out of this neurotoxicity."[64]

Among the items of continuing research was a 2017 study, which concluded that artificially sweetened soft drink consumption was associated with a higher risk of stroke and dementia.[65]

Nonetheless, artificial sweeteners remain a sweet favorite of the food industry. Millions of consumers, battling obesity and hoping to curb their sugar consumption, use tabletop sweeteners and eat artificially sweetened foods.

* * *

In summary, our food system is now largely composed of genetically engineered and nutritionally bankrupt foods or food-like substances, laced with a staggering array of pesticides, herbicides, GMOs, artificial sweeteners, colors, and flavors, and a host of chemicals. These are linked to inflammation and compromising the proper functioning of our bodies with consequences for our long-term health.

While today's modern diet may provide beneficial protection from micro- and macro-nutrient deficiencies, our overabundance of calories and the macronutrients that compose our diet may all lead to increased inflammation, reduced control of infection, increased rates of cancer, and increased risk for allergic and auto-inflammatory disease.[66]

Ian A. Myles, nutritional expert

Hormone Imbalances

Hormones are chemical messengers that coordinate complex processes involved in many functions, like growth, metabolism, appetite, sleep, fertility, immunity, and behavior. In responding to signals from the brain, hormones are secreted directly into the blood by the glands that produce and store them. These glands form a network known as the endocrine system. While all cells are exposed to hormones circulating in the bloodstream, only the ones which have receptors for that hormone will respond to its signal. When a hormone binds to its receptor, it causes a biological response.

Chemicals that interfere with the function of hormones are identified as endocrine disruptors. They can act at any point along this hormone signaling pathway, causing such disruptions as blocking it from binding to its receptor or being synthesized. Disturbances in any of these hormones can influence the way your brain functions and lead to imbalances resulting in many different conditions, e.g., depression, dementia, anxiety, weight loss, weight gain, and obesity.[67]

Sedentary Lifestyles

> *Physical exercise is one of the most potent ways of changing your genes; put simply, when you exercise, your literally exercise your genes. Aerobic exercise in particular not only turns on genes linked to longevity, but also targets the BDNF gene, the brain's "growth hormone."* [68]
> David Perlmutter, MD

Exercise is well known to reduce inflammation with powerful effects upon the brain. Likewise, a sedentary lifestyle is detrimental to health and is connected to the progression of all the most common neurodegenerative conditions.[69]

When you move, your muscle cells release a small protein called Interleukin 6, or IL-6, which research reveals fights inflammation during exercise. This has several anti-inflammatory effects, including lowering levels of a protein called TNF alpha, which itself triggers inflammation in the body.[70]

Exercise has been shown to increase BDNF, "brain-derived neurotrophic factor," which plays a key role in creating new neurons and important for neurogenesis, the process by which new neurons are formed in the brain. Decreased levels of BDNF are associated with psychiatric and neurological conditions.[71]

Age is linked to rising levels of chronic inflammation, so staying active and exercising are very beneficial for keeping it at bay.

Sleep

Although we value the joy of sound sleep, many of us are often challenged to enjoy adequate, restorative sleep. After age 60, nighttime sleep tends to be shorter, lighter, and interrupted by multiple awakenings. Medications can also interfere with sleep.

Sleep is critical to the brain, including how nerve cells (neurons) communicate with each other. Disrupted or insufficient sleep can cause a rise in cortisol leading to many health issues, ranging from depression, dementia, and reduced immune function to weight gain and other chronic conditions.[72]

"Poor sleep may be a risk factor for Alzheimer's," says Professor Benca, who conducted a 2015 research study of 98 participants without dementia. "Recent findings suggest that during sleep, toxins that build up while you are awake, including beta amyloid and tau proteins, implicated in their connection to Alzheimer's, are removed from your brain."[73]

Chronic Infections

In summary, the organisms that live within us—those that constitute our holobiome (the sum total of microbiomes of our gut, skin, sinuses, etc.) and those that invade and infect us—are critical determinants of our cognition, risk for cognitive decline, and progression of cognitive decline. [74]

Dale Bredesen, MD

Inflammation accompanies an infection. When the body detects pathogens, the immune system responds in many ways. Inflammation is a "second defense" against a tissue injury such as from an environmental agent, toxic chemical, or infection. When inflammation is present in the body, there will be higher levels of substances known as biomarkers.[75] Specific biomarkers help doctors identify the presence or severity of inflammation and may test for specific inflammatory markers such as C-reactive protein (CRP), homocysteine, MMP9, TNF alpha, and others specific to a suspected agent.

Note: See chapter 20, "Smart Choices in Today's Toxic Times," for lifestyle recommendations and interventions to help reduce or prevent this destructive process.

Chapter 15
The Rise of Autoimmune Issues

The lack of knowledge and awareness surrounding autoimmunity results in untold suffering for people affected by these diseases. Misdiagnosis and delayed diagnosis can result in damage to vital organs.[1]

The Autoimmune Association

After Rick was diagnosed with the autoimmune disease, toxic encephalopathy, it was time for me to learn more about autoimmunity. It occurs when your immune system, which defends your body against disease, decides your healthy cells are foreign invaders. As a result, your immune system attacks your healthy cells and releases autoantibodies, triggering an inflammatory response.

An autoimmune disease can affect one or many different types of body tissues and destroy them.[2] Although one part of the body may be targeted such as in diabetes which affects the pancreas, autoimmune diseases often have a multi-symptom, multi-systemic impact. For instance, while Type 1 diabetes attacks the pancreas it also affects the eyes, glands, muscles, kidneys and more. In Rick's case with his diagnosis of toxic encephalopathy, an autoimmune disorder, an explosion of symptoms flared up throughout his body as well as his brain.

In the late 1980's, prior to Rick's illness, I began learning of unusual conditions that were being diagnosed by doctors in some of my friends, as well as some of Rick's clients.

- In 1987, Suzanne, our neighbor in northern Virginia, was diagnosed with fibromyalgia. She said that explained the collection of symptoms she had noticed for some time and complained about regularly—her constant bout with muscle aches, pains, difficulty sleeping, GI issues, headaches, and sheer exhaustion.

- Not long afterwards, friend Michelle announced she had been diagnosed with Hashimoto's thyroiditis. She shared how her active life had been transformed—she was losing clumps of hair, gaining weight, and feeling drop-dead fatigued. The condition was also linked to her difficulty in getting pregnant and several miscarriages.

- A few months later, during an outing with my daughter's Girl Scout troop, Alyssa (one of the chaperone mothers) told of the symptoms associated with her recently diagnosed lupus. Among her problems: she was depressed; drained of energy; had red, blotchy rashes; and experienced horrible GI issues. Although often feeling sick and exhausted, she was fighting hard to keep up with her family's activities.

Until these encounters, I had never met anyone previously who had been diagnosed with such a collection of symptoms, now recognized as autoimmune in nature. I wondered what was causing an increasing number of unusual cases with many similar symptoms.

A recent review of literature concluded that worldwide rates of rheumatic, endocrinological, gastrointestinal, and neurological autoimmune diseases are increasing by 4 to 7% per year ... and the greatest increases are occurring in countries in the Northern and Western Hemispheres.[3]

Geoff Rutledge, MD, PhD

Indeed, the incidence of autoimmune diseases is increasing at an alarming rate. But are these diseases really rising, or are doctors now becoming more educated regarding their symptoms and therefore able to diagnose patients more effectively? Dr. Rutledge explains, "It is true that as we broaden the definitions of autoimmune disease, and as more people learn about these conditions, more people are diagnosed. We also have more sensitive lab tests that detect autoimmune conditions that are not yet symptomatic."[4]

As of mid-2021, the Autoimmune Association estimates that at least 100 different autoimmune diseases currently exist.[5] While the National Institutes of Health (NIH) estimates about 23.5 million Americans suffer from autoimmune diseases, the Autoimmune Association states that these diseases afflict more than 50 million people. The difference between numbers is that NIH only includes 24 diseases for which good epidemiology studies are available.[6]

So why are so many people wrestling with these debilitating diseases? Research in the conventional medicine community confirms at least two contributing factors: genetics and environment issues. "Virtually every autoimmune disease combines these two," writes Dr. Noel R. Rose, who is recognized as the 'father of autoimmunology. "In autoimmune disease, multiple genes are involved; we have genes that collectively increase the vulnerability or susceptibility to autoimmune disease. What is inherited is not a specific gene that causes a specific defect in metabolism; several genes increase vulnerability or susceptibility to autoimmune disease."[7]

As described in *The Autoimmune Epidemic: Bodies Gone Haywire in a World out of Balance*: "But for those with a genetic vulnerability to autoimmunity, even a small dose [of toxic exposure] may trigger disease, creating a cellular mayhem in which the body begins to destroy its own blood, tissue, nerves and organs. And this is what concerns researchers the most. For those 25% of people around the world who do have a genetic predisposition to autoimmunity, it may not take very much exposure to cause cells to miscommunicate."[8] This miscommunication leads to autoimmunity.

According to the Autoimmune Association, "a close genetic relationship exists among autoimmune disease, explaining clustering in individuals and families as well as a common pathway of disease."[9] This does not mean family members will manifest the same autoimmune disease. Rather, they share a tendency toward autoimmunity, which may express itself in differing diseases.

"Genes are not a diagnosis; genes are just potential," says Robin Berzin, MD. "So we have to look at what is turning on the genes."[10] And, largely, it's environment and the impact of what happens biochemically within the genetically susceptible as to how that triggers or turns on those genes to express themselves.

Fortunately, the science of *epigenetics* is uncovering answers and helping researchers understand the connection between disease and heredity in a variety of human disorders and fatal diseases. Epigenetics is the study of changes in organisms caused by modification of gene expression—physical traits or biochemical characteristics based on a combination of genes and environmental factors—as opposed to the alteration of the genetic code of the cell, the genotype. By understanding the epigenetic mechanisms, researchers can develop therapeutic strategies to manipulate immune regulation.

The Autoimmunity Centers of Excellence (ACEs) was created to encourage research for improving the lives of patients with autoimmune diseases by assisting them with better diagnosis, clinical trial design, therapeutic development, and treatment selection. Funding for the research is provided from grants by the National Institute of Allergy and Infectious Diseases.[11]

More research is vital to understanding the autoimmune process. As Dr. Rose stated in 2019: "It is going to be, I think, an equally fascinating chapter in the saga of autoimmune disease in the next decade."[12] Recognizing the complex nature of human disease and the environment, Dr. Judith Stern makes the analogy: "Genetics loads the gun, but environment pulls the trigger."[13]

Our Genetic Roulette Wheel

Through Rick's illness, I learned about his genetic link to autoimmune issues and chronic inflammatory illnesses, which spurred me to find out if our daughters carried genes with similar potential. I needed to know if they had inherited Rick's "dreaded genotype," a phrase coined by Dr. Ritchie Shoemaker to describe a genotype carried by approximately 2% of the population which compromises full recovery. I was also curious to see what my genetic profile might reveal.

Fortunately, our daughters do not have Rick's rare haplotype (HLA), but to my surprise they share similar genetics from my side of the family. Although neither our daughters nor myself were manifesting any symptoms, I wanted the information added to our health histories going forward.

Our family medical history was becoming clearer. My brother had been diagnosed years earlier with polymyositis, an autoimmune condition that fortunately resolved itself.

The Visual Contrast Sensitivity (VCS) screening test I had taken at Dr. Shoemaker's office indicated I had issues that needed further evaluation. Maybe those occasional bouts of sinus infections and a few cases of bronchitis were related to biotoxins?

From additional testing of my genetics, I learned I was also a poor detoxifier.

I followed through with Shoemaker's protocol for detoxification and developed a habit of regularly detoxing using an herbal cleanse. With my attention focused on the care of both Rick and my mother, I did not pursue follow-up testing to see whether the biotoxins had fully cleared.

After my mother had moved into our basement, she developed sinus infections, multiple bouts of bronchitis and pneumonia, and her arthritis worsened. Her mainstream medical team attributed her symptoms to her age, and prescribed steroids to treat her inflammatory reactions.

Since my mother was then in her 80s, I did not question the connection between her increasing health problems and her age. However, while reading Dr. Ritchie Shoemaker's book, *Mold Warriors*, to learn more about Rick's toxicity issues, I connected Mom's maladies to a possible genetic susceptibility for autoimmune disorders. A trip to the Eastern Shore to have her evaluated at the CRBAI confirmed Mom had the HLA haplotype that made her a poor detoxifier and more vulnerable for autoimmune illnesses like her rheumatoid arthritis.

My mother's medical team had treated her symptoms with steroids, and as Dr. Shoemaker notes in *Mold Warriors:* "Treating biotoxin illnesses with steroids is similar to 'throwing gasoline on a fire,' and with good reasons. I can't tell you how many biotoxin disasters I've seen, from optic neuritis being turned into blindness to inflammatory joints turning into frozen joints when a physician prescribed steroids. Don't let anyone give them to you if you're biotoxic!"[14]

Naturally, I would prefer if my daughters and I were not genetically prone to autoimmune conditions, but this information is especially critical for us to be aware of the risks associated with environmental exposures and other inflammatory triggers.

The Mighty Microbiome

One of those risks is associated with nurturing the microbiome since imbalances can trigger inflammatory reactions, leading to autoimmune conditions. In 2007, the National Institutes of Health launched the Human Microbiome Project to study the collective genomes of the bacteria, fungi, protozoa viruses, and other microbes that live inside and on the human body. This groundbreaking research opened a portal of continuing discoveries about this interconnected pathway and the links to health.

The trillions of microbes collectively known as the microbiome play multiple roles—digesting food to generate nutrients for cells, synthesizing vitamins, metabolizing drugs, detoxifying carcinogens, stimulating renewal of cells in the gut lining, developing neurons, and activating and supporting the immune system. A healthy GI system needs healthy, good bacteria.[15]

The gut microbiome is impacted by your genes, your immune system, infections, antibiotic use, and what you eat and drink, among other factors that influence the diversity of your gut's microbiota. When studies evaluate diet and the gut microbiota, they review the diversity of bacteria—a low diversity can cause issues; as well as having too much of others. For instance, if the good gut bacteria are compromised, this may lead to a yeast infection, particularly one known as *candida albicans*, a fungus found in mucous membranes. When yeast is maintained in appropriate levels in the body, it helps with nutrient absorption and digestion. However, when there is an overgrowth of bacteria, yeast, and fungi, this can unleash a condition known as dysbiosis.

Beyond causing intestinal distress with characteristic gas and bloating, dysbiosis interferes with food digestion and delivery of important nutrients needed by the body. It can also lead to a wide range of issues, including leaky gut, periodontal (gum) disease, oral thrush, sinus infections, mood disorders, vaginal and urinary tract infections, and others. It has been linked to a wide range of conditions, including inflammatory bowel disease (IBD), obesity, allergic disorders, Type 1 diabetes mellitus, autism, liver disease, dementia, and colorectal cancer, in both human and animal models.[16] These are complex disorders with many causes, yet the gut microbiome is central to them all.

If the immune system is compromised, candida can migrate to other parts of the body, including the brain and heart. The toxins produced by the yeast and other bacteria stimulate the immune system and fire cytokines, the body's infection-fighting agents. When excess cytokines are produced, they can attack tissues and cells, leading to increased inflammation, autoimmunity, and brain issues.[17]

Research has recently linked oral bacteria, specifically, *Porphyromonas gingivalis*, the bacteria present in the most serious form of gum disease, to Alzheimer's. Bacteria can travel from the mouth to the brain, creating toxins called *gingipains*, which cause damage to human proteins and destroy brain cells and nerves.[18]

Prior to Rick's total health collapse in 2004, he was regularly being treated for periodontal disease. This was years before science recognized the connection between the oral microbiome and brain issues. Bacteria and abscesses in the mouth and other hidden infections can cause gut dysfunction, triggering the potential for autoimmune diseases, especially in those who are genetically prone. While Rick was in the throes of his GI issues, I was unaware of any connection to how dental disease may have contributed to his illness, nor were any of his doctors.

Leaky Guts and Leaky Brains

Restoring the microbiome is key to efficient immune function. Microbiome research is currently one of the hottest areas of medical exploration with scientists seeking clues as to how the trillion-cell ecosystem of microbes living inside and on our bodies impacts our health.

Microbiome researchers see the gut as ground zero for autoimmune havoc. An estimated 70-80% of the body's immune cells are found in the gut, where bacteria regulate the immune system.[19] The mouth, the first step in the digestive process, has its own oral microbiome, and science now recognizes that dental infections can have a huge impact on overall health. (See chapter 17, in the section, "A Mouthful of Mercury and More.")

Our microbiomes are literally being assaulted with antibiotics, painkillers, prescription medications, and all the refined and processed foods, sugars, and gluten that have become standard American fare. This abuse upsets the gut's natural microbiota diversity and can trigger intestinal permeability, known as "leaky gut." The term describes the passing of material from inside the gastrointestinal tract through the cells lining the gut wall, and into the bloodstream.[20]

Normally, the intestine allows some permeability through a very thin barrier so nutrients can pass through the gut, while keeping out potentially harmful, foreign substances from leaving the intestine and traveling outside the digestive system. However, with a leaky gut, cell damage can make that barrier porous, allowing harmful substances to pass into the bloodstream, activating the immune system and ramping up inflammation.

While leaky gut syndrome is recognized by some conventional practitioners, others in mainstream medicine view it only as a hypothetical condition. In contrast, functional medicine links leaky gut syndrome to chronic inflammation and the onset of autoimmune disorders, certain types of cancer, fatty liver conditions, and schizophrenia, among other diseases.[21]

The brain has its own protective lining, known as the blood-brain barrier (BBB) to keep harmful chemicals, heavy metals, toxins, infectious pathogens, and wayward immune cells away from the brain. To function properly, the brain must be supplied with glucose, amino acids, and fat-soluble nutrients among others, delivered via the semi-permeable blood vessels into the brain.[22] This is one way the blood-brain barrier is penetrated by harmful trespassers, igniting neuroinflammation. This can result in brain fog, depression, anxiety, and a host of neurodegenerative diseases, including dementia, Parkinson's, and Alzheimer's.[23]

Functional medicine recognizes the triad of genetic predisposition, environmental triggers that turn on the genes, and intestinal permeability must all be present to develop an autoimmune disease and is at the forefront of autoimmune disease research. While we cannot change our genes, we can reduce our exposure to environmental triggers and address our intestinal permeability by supporting a healthy microbiome in our gut. "With its focus on understanding each individual's unique genetics and environment—and the interactions between them—as well as its longstanding appreciation of the importance of the microbiome and intestinal permeability, Functional Medicine is perfectly positioned to help patients prevent and reverse autoimmune diseases."[24]

Conventional medical science believes once autoimmune diseases are triggered by a combination of genetics and environmental toxicity, the process cannot be reversed. However, research by Alessio Fasano, MD—founder and director of the Center for Celiac Research at Massachusetts General Hospital—has discovered that by removing the intestinal permeability issue and/or the trigger, an autoimmune condition will go into remission: "If we're able to stop the autoimmune process, an entire world of possibilities opens for treating autoimmune diseases for which there are currently no solutions."[25]

Functional medicine recognizes that nutritional supplements, probiotics, herbal remedies, and special diets (i.e., gluten-free, antifungal, low sugar) can be pivotal in healing leaky gut syndrome.

Food Sensitivities

Food sensitivities can cause and perpetuate a leaky gut. As more people are experiencing digestive distress often linked to gluten and dairy, they are seeking plant-based and gluten-free options. However, the list of potential food triggers is more extensive and can include nuts, seeds, eggs, and members of the nightshade family (potatoes, tomatoes, bell peppers, eggplant, and others).

Soy is another food that can cause problems for some, especially when it's genetically modified, which currently accounts for about 95% of soy production. Soy contains phytoestrogens (estrogen mimickers) and can cause hormone imbalances in those who are sensitive.[26]

Rick was never tested for food sensitivities, so I cannot confirm if this was a factor, but he did have a penchant for sugar, which is highly inflammatory to the gut. During his years of residence in hospitals, nursing homes, and assisted living facilities, Rick consumed a highly processed, starchy, sugar-filled diet. It is a sad fact that in many hospitals and nursing facilities, patients are fed these types of diet, which are inflammatory by nature.

Over the years, Rick was also on multiple rounds of antibiotics for periodontitis, a bacterial infection of candida, and his post-hernia surgery, suspected Lyme disease and multiple urinary tract infections. This may also have triggered small intestinal bacterial overgrowth (SIBO), a condition caused by antibiotic overuse and starchy foods. SIBO increases intestinal permeability as the body attempts to purge the excess bacteria from the gut.[27]

According to functional medicine, increased intestinal permeability usually develops prior to the onset of disease, and is associated with a variety of triggers as detailed by Izabella Wentz in her book, *Hashimoto's Thyroiditis—Lifestyle Interventions for Finding and Treating the Root Cause*:[28]

- Food intolerances
- Stress
- Poor digestion
- Nonsteroidal anti-inflammatory drugs (NSAIDS)
- Alcohol
- Enzyme deficiencies

- Infections

- Nutrient deficiencies (especially in fatty acids, amino acids, zinc and glutamine)

- Imbalance of gut flora

Functional medicine upholds the belief that optimizing gut function is one of the crucial steps for optimizing the immune system. After struggling with symptoms for years, Dr. Wentz was able to reverse her own decade-long bout with Hashimoto's disease.

It was once believed that after the autoimmune process is activated, it becomes independent of continuous exposure to the environmental trigger, resulting in a self-sustain and irreversible cycle. However, examples of autoimmune recovery have discredited the "irreversible" aspect of this theory. It has been shown that continuous environmental triggers are necessary to perpetuate the process. This means the autoimmune process can be stopped and reversed when the triggers are eliminated.[29]

Izabella Wentz, PharmD, FASCP

Chapter 16
Gut Issues—Ground Zero for Inflammation

Your gut microbes are engaged in ongoing conversations with your GI tract, your immune system, your enteric nervous system, and your brain—and as with any cooperative relationship, healthy communication is essential. Recent research reveals that the disturbance of these conversations can lead to GI diseases ... and may be involved in the development of many serious brain diseases, including depression, Alzheimer's disease, and autism.[1]

Emeran Mayer, MD

Prior to the onslaught of his illness, Rick did not complain much about any digestive issues, but he would frequently pop antacids, often belching loudly at times. The girls and I thought it was just an annoying habit. Back then, I was not tracking any of the interconnections between the gut and brain.

During Rick's first hospitalization in March 2004, a CT scan did not indicate any issues with his organs. However, his GI issues intensified over time, including constipation and heartburn, as well as unrelenting abdominal pain becoming unbearable. "My stomach hurts!" became his chronic call for help.

I arranged for a consultation with a gastroenterologist, who ordered an endoscopy to investigate problems in Rick's stomach and esophagus. It revealed only minor inflammation. The specialist prescribed Rick a daily medication to reduce his stomach acid, but it didn't help much. In recent discussions with functional doctors, I've learned that many prescriptions and over-the-counter antacid medications can be detrimental to the gastrointestinal tract. Overuse can also contribute to aluminum toxicity and cause electrolyte imbalances.

The gastroenterologist also scheduled a colonoscopy to explore Rick's lower GI tract. Again, it revealed nothing unusual. Because his gut issues continued to be unresolved, I arranged for another consultation. Based on Rick's continuing discomfort, the gastroenterologist suspected gastroparesis, a condition in which the stomach does not empty itself of food so it can move through the digestive system. The food then ferments in the stomach and can lead to bacterial growth. Medications, including narcotics and antidepressants, are linked to this condition; Rick's doctors prescribed plenty of them to manage both his neurological and pain issues.

When I asked one how they would confirm this condition, he said, "We do a test using radioactive eggs, which trace his digestion."

"And if it's positive, then what?" I asked.

The doctor replied, "We give him medication to treat the symptoms. There isn't really a cure and with all his current medications, and your concern about his toxicity, a new medication would only be adding to it."

I agreed. Dumping more toxins into a man already burdened with a heavy toxic load did not seem wise. Toxins stimulate cytokine production, which can in turn trigger inflammatory reactions in the central nervous system and the autonomic nervous system. This interferes with intestinal motility, slowing down digestion and the elimination process.

The following week I consulted with one of Rick's integrative health professionals about his digestive issues. I was now shuttling Rick between conventional and integrative doctors in hopes one or the other would offer a beneficial treatment plan. His naturopathic doctor recommended a multi-enzyme at meals to improve his digestion and to make yogurt part of his regular diet. None of the gastroenterologists we consulted ever mentioned giving him a probiotic, a multi-enzyme supplement, or even yogurt. It was encouraging that shortly after starting Rick on this regimen, his GI issues improved.

When I asked Rick's conventional doctors why he suffered from so much digestive distress, they all echoed the same explanation—"nervous stomachs" are associated with anxiety, stress, worry, and neurotic or psychiatric issues, all which Rick displayed.

In defense of his doctors, Rick's sudden health collapse preceded the groundbreaking research that revealed the interconnections of the gut, brain, and microbiome. Science would soon demonstrate (but not soon enough for Rick) that an imbalanced gut microbiome is linked to brain issues—depression, panic disorders, anxiety, dementia, and autism.

It was only after Rick's death in 2016, when I read *The Mind-Gut Connection* by Emeran Mayer, that I would learn how vital a healthy gut is to both preventing and healing chronic illnesses, especially those related to brain issues. Rick's habit of loudly belching was a signal of the inflammatory process stirring up problems. No one at the time mentioned any connection that a healthy gut is fundamental not only to brain health, but for proper functioning of the whole body.

It turns out that the protein that clumps to form Lewy bodies, alpha-synuclein, exists not only in patients' brains, but also in nerve cells within their gut. In fact, certain nerve cells in the enteric nervous system degenerate years before other Parkinson's symptoms appear, compromising the elaborate functioning of the little brain in the gut, slowing peristalsis, and delaying the transit of stool through the colon.[2]

Emeran Mayer, MD

The Vital Connection of the Gut-Brain Axis

The vagus nerve allows for two-way communication between the brain and internal organs, including the heart, lungs, and digestive tract. In addition to an intricate communications network, the gut has its own nervous system, called the enteric nervous system (ENS). The gut and brain are also linked by chemicals called neurotransmitters, such as serotonin, some of which are produced in other organs, not exclusively in the brain as scientists once believed.[3]

About 95% of serotonin, the chemical that helps regulate mood, happiness, and feelings of well-being, is produced by the gut's nerve cells.[4] So when the gut is not functioning well, it is not surprising that those with digestive issues manifest depressive symptoms.

As science expands its understanding of the gut-brain connection and the role microbes contribute to mood and mental health, revolutionary therapies are being envisioned for treating brain-related disorders by altering the microbiome. Researchers Michael Toh and Emma Allen-Vercoe note the critical connection of the microbiome to brain health:

> "The human gut-microbiota is a complex microbial ecosystem that contributes an important component towards the health of its host. This highly complex ecosystem has been underestimated in its importance until recently, when a realization of the enormous scope of gut microbiota function has been (and continues to be) revealed. One of the more striking of these discoveries is the finding that the gut microbiota and the brain are connected, and thus there is potential for the microbiota in the gut to influence behavior and mental health."[5]

For those of us with cognitive decline, or at risk for cognitive decline, the status of our gut microbiomes—the makeup of the various bacteria and other microbes in our intestines—is critical, since the human gut microbiome plays an important role in virtually all of the major risk factors and drivers of cognitive decline: inflammation, autoimmunity, insulin resistance, lipid metabolism, obesity, nutrient absorption, amyloidogenesis, * *neurochemistry, sleep, stress response, and detoxification.*[6]

Dale Bredesen, MD

---

*Amyloidogenesis is the formation or growth of amyloid structures, linked to Alzheimer's disease, Parkinson's disease, type II diabetes, and others.
Source: https://www.ncbi.nlm.nih.gov/medgen/317372

Chapter 17
Neurotoxicity—Toxic Assault of the Brain

It is not unusual for patients suffering from neurotoxicity to be misdiagnosed as having psychological problems because of their anxiety and depression levels, their sheer number of symptoms and their belief that chemicals made them ill.[1]

Dr. Raymond Singer

While Rick's illness seemed like a medical aberration, his case reflected many similar symptoms increasingly diagnosed in other patients. He was just one of millions suffering from exhaustion, anxiety, depression, brain fog, delusions, hallucinations, seizures, and other neurological issues. Unfortunately, patients treated in conventional medicine are often given a diagnosis, but never fully evaluated for the organic, underlying causes.

When psychiatrists overlook the connection between mental issues and imbalances in other bodily systems—e.g., toxic overload, gut function, the immune system, and hormones—it is easy to miss the underlying causes of neurodegeneration.

Mitochondrial cell damage is at the heart of neurodegeneration. It plays a significant role in the pathogenesis of a wide range of seemingly unrelated disorders, including schizophrenia, bipolar issues, dementias, epilepsy, migraines, neuropathic pain, Parkinson's disease, chronic fatigue syndrome, fibromyalgia, and other chronic conditions. Medications are linked to mitochondrial damage, including all classes of psychotropic drugs, statin medications, and analgesics, such as acetaminophen and others.[2]

Too often physicians practice what Dr. Paul McHugh (a psychiatrist, researcher, and professor) referred to as "DSM checklist psychiatry," with the goal of achieving a diagnosis rather than inquiring deeply into the sources and nature of an affliction."[3]

I believe Rick was a victim of "DSM checklist psychiatry," as he was repeatedly evaluated by various teams of psychiatrists who believed his condition was psychiatric rather than a result of neurotoxicity, which manifests similar symptoms. I continually provided Rick's full history of chemical, heavy metals, and biotoxin exposures, but that information was generally dismissed.

In their article, "Recognizing Neurotoxicity," Dr. Raymond Singer and Dana Darby Johnson clearly describe the complex nature of neurotoxic impact upon patients. As a neurotoxic forensic expert witness, Dr. Singer's insights would have highlighted the issues that doctors were not properly testing for—or overlooking.

It is an excellent resource that I only wish I had discovered at the time to share with Rick's treating physicians. It is an excellent resource and recommended reading especially if you are exploring possibilities for unexplained symptoms and behaviors.[4] I encourage you to refer to Appendix A.

Neurotoxicity patients may well have psychological problems, but these are often the result, not the cause, of their condition.

Dr. Raymond Singer

Chemical Connections

Fortunately, Rev. Lowell Smith, our trusted friend of 30 years, offered his unwavering support throughout our 12-year journey. As a long-time friend, he was a guiding light through our valleys of despair. We were grateful for his wisdom in many arenas, which yielded new insights.

In addition to being a caring man of great love and wisdom, Lowell was an MIT graduate in electrical engineering, with knowledge of chemicals, heavy metals, and their impact upon health. Tanning leather is one of the most toxic industries in the world because of the chemicals involved.[5] Once he became aware of the toxic nature of Rick's environment years earlier, Lowell suggested their possible connection. As we would learn, with Rick's genetics as a poor detoxifier, toxins accumulate in the body and serve as inflammatory agents triggering many imbalances.

Rick's long-term, chemical exposure was never considered as a potential factor in his illness. Years before his illness, while visiting his boyhood home and the leather tannery, he told our daughters that (as I mentioned in chapter 13) as a child a favorite pastime was jumping into the tanned hides for fun. How he loved the smell of tanned leather! Additionally, his turn-of-the-century home adjacent to his father's leather tanning factory contained lead pipes and lead paint.

High levels of toxic metals deposited in body tissues and subsequently in the brain can cause significant developmental and neurological damage. Toxic metals do not have any useful physiological function, adversely affect almost every organ system, and disrupt homeostasis, the equilibrium in the body.[6]

Chemicals, biotoxins, and heavy metals—directly or indirectly—impact the brain and have been overlooked all too often. The feature, "Toxins and Infections," which appears on the website of the Neuro-Luminance Brain Health Centers reinforces their connection: "Just as the long-term impact of

Traumatic Brain Injury was downplayed for many, many years, the impact of toxins and infections upon brain function have been downplayed and ridiculed as hysteria."[7]

As reported by Dr. Keith Berndtson in his comprehensive "Chronic Inflammatory Response Syndrome—Overview, Diagnosis and Treatment" monograph, toxins are drawn to tissues with rich nerve supplies, and the brain appears to be a common target. Dr. Berndtson writes, "Due to their small size, ionophore neurotoxins may gain easy entry into the brain, perhaps more easily in the presence of weak spots in the blood-brain barrier."[8]

Chelation Treatments for Removing Heavy Metals

In June 2004, with recognition of Rick's history of chemical exposures, I scheduled an appointment for Rick with a well-known internist in the DC suburbs who specialized in chelation treatments. Chelation therapy is an intravenous treatment using EDTA (ethylenediamine tetraacetic acid), which bonds with the heavy metals, enabling their excretion through urine. Although not without its risks, chelation therapy is an effective way to detox heavy metals, so many doctors recommend this treatment if there is moderate to severe heavy metal poisoning.

The internist ordered a 24-hour provoked urine test, to get an accurate baseline reading on Rick's toxic load, It revealed very high levels of lead, cadmium, and aluminum, along with other toxic metals, including mercury. The doctor suggested he start with ten chelation treatments, and then re-test again to see if Rick's high numbers had improved.

EDTA is approved by the Food and Drug Administration for treating lead poisoning and high calcium levels and is used in both conventional and integrative medicine to remove heavy metals. While the benefits of EDTA chelation for lead poisoning and removing high levels of calcium is undisputed, medical supervision is vital.[9]

Rick and I trekked weekly to the Virginia countryside for his infusions, a combination of EDTA, vitamins, minerals, and glutathione, a critical antioxidant needed for detoxification. The treatments lasted about three hours and were not covered by insurance. Yet, judging from the rooms packed with patients attached to intravenous drips, many believed in the power of chelation treatments!

I engaged in some chairside chats with other patients during these treatments. Most reported that their heavy-metals-provoked urine tests initially indicated high levels of mercury and lead, and that they were undergoing treatment to remove these dangerous toxins.

After ten chelation treatments, the doctors repeated Rick's urine test. Unfortunately, his numbers barely budged. The internist supervising chelation treatments could not tell me with confidence that Rick's numbers would improve, even with an additional 20, 30, or 40 more treatments.

Unfortunately, these treatments and lab tests were all out-of-pocket expenses and with our financial burdens mounting, I suspended them—a decision I later regretted. It was only after his death, when I was undergoing my own chelation treatments for high lead and aluminum readings, that I learned readings from the first ten treatments may not reflect much movement.

In retrospect, I should have committed to more treatments. At least I could have seen whether they would have changed outcomes. Back then, I did not have clarity about chelation and what it would require to lighten Rick's toxic load.

In dealing with a condition not well-recognized or validated by Rick's conventional doctors, I had to rely on my own intuition and piece-meal information I uncovered along the way. I was not always certain of my abilities to discern the right path, a struggle I encountered many times. As I would learn later, Rick's issues were not just from heavy metals and chemical exposure, but also from biotoxins, which required a different form of detoxification. At any rate, releasing the accumulation of his lifetime exposures was challenging for his genetically ill-equipped body.

In seeking treatments throughout the first two years of Rick's illness, several different doctors from both conventional and integrative practices conducted heavy metals testing. From both urine collections and hair sample tests conducted in integrative practices, Rick scored high in lead, chromium, arsenic, aluminum, mercury, uranium, and other metals. His hair sample report stated that "clinical research indicates that hair levels of specific elements, particularly potentially toxic elements such as cadmium, mercury, lead and arsenic, are highly correlated with pathological disorders." His urine test confirmed similar results.

The symptoms associated with heavy metal toxicity aligned with Rick's own: mental confusion; pain, swelling, and stiffness in muscles and joints; numbness and tingling in extremities; headaches; short-term memory loss; gastrointestinal issues; vision problems; chronic fatigue; drowsiness; depression and mood swings; neuritis; poor concentration; and impulsive, unpredictable behavior. Heavy metals testing certainly seemed to nail what Rick was experiencing.

These insights provided new dimensions for the benefit of our family and friends with new awareness of what likely had contributed to his symptoms. Not surprisingly, this information was not considered by his conventional treatment teams, yet I remained hopeful that a medical professional somewhere in our consultations would validate this connection.

Defining Differences in Toxic Metals Testing

There are significant differences in toxic metals testing and protocols for what and how to test. Blood or hair testing for heavy metal toxicity reveals acute metal poisoning, which is rare. These tests do not measure the heavy metal burden accumulated over a lifetime of exposure. Heavy metals have a short half-life in the blood; they then move into tissues for storage. Hence, a blood analysis is not indicative of the actual level in the body and why a provoked urine test is needed.[10]

Sherry A. Rogers, MD, author of *Detoxify or Die*, states "People do not stock-pile much of their heavy metals in their blood cells, but they have lots hidden in the brain, kidneys, and bones or in some other important target organ like the heart. You cannot use blood tests to measure metal loads. The only way to find heavy metals is to do a heavy metal provocation test."[11]

An accurate, objective analysis, known as a metal mobilization test (MMT) can only be obtained by administering a metal chelating agent that pulls heavy metals from tissues and releases them into the urine. Proper assessment is critical in assessing chronic illnesses, especially regarding cognitive issues, neurological conditions, immune dysfunction, and depression.[12]

Since Rick's heavy metals exposure was long-term rather than acute, his blood tests did not reveal anything alarming. His allopathic neurologist reported that his bloodwork was well within the range, so she discounted any consideration of heavy metal toxicity. Provoked urine testing offers valuable insights, yet no standards exist for its testing and remains controversial.

I wish I had known at the time that there were distinct differences in testing for heavy metals. At the time, I still had faith in the wisdom of conventional medicine, and not yet fully confident in integrative practices. Over the course of Rick's illness, my confidence in the integrative model of medicine would dramatically shift.

A Mouthful of Mercury and More

Adverse health effects from mercury exposure include: tremors, impaired vision and hearing, paralysis, insomnia, emotional instability, developmental deficits during fetal development, and attention deficit and developmental delays during childhood. Recent studies suggest that mercury may have no threshold below which some adverse effects do not occur. [13]

World Health Organization

Throughout the dozen years of Rick's illness, no conventional medical or dental evaluation ever considered how Rick's dental issues may also have contributed to his illness—from mercury exposure from his mouthful of dental amalgams to the bacterial infection from his pre-existing periodontitis.

Peering into Rick's mouth usually accompanied his many medical exams, but no physicians noted anything significant until November 2007, three years after he fell ill. In preparing for Rick's release from the state mental hospital, a dental exam revealed he had seven abscessed teeth. (After six months residing at the hospital, they just discovered he had seven abscessed teeth!?)

Prior to the onset of his illness, Rick was being treated for periodontal (gum) disease. This was perhaps before science recognized the connection between bleeding gums/gingivitis and bacteria traveling from the mouth to the brain. Groundbreaking research now links imbalances of mouth microbes to chronic illness including diabetes, cancer, and dementia.[14]

Rick's mouth, full of amalgams, inflamed and bleeding gums, and perhaps even a failed root canal or two, presented additional avenues for toxic and bacterial invasion of his body and brain. Extracting his seven abscessed teeth opened more risks for infection from the exposed holes in his gums.

Researchers have measured brain mercury levels in people with mercury amalgam fillings and discovered that the levels are disproportionately higher in those with twelve or more dental fillings. He had at least a "dirty dozen" of amalgam fillings.

The body's natural mechanism to rid itself of mercury is compromised as the blood-brain membrane becomes saturated; once that happens, higher doses of mercury remain inside the brain. Unfortunately, mainstream practitioners and conventional dentists did not examine Rick's mercury levels, so another piece of his toxic body burden was missed.

As Neil Nathan, MD, relates in his book, *Toxic*, "Even minuscule amounts of mercury can poison the key enzyme of methylation, methionine synthase, which works with methyl cobalamin (vitamin B_{12}) to convert homocysteine to methionine. This severely compromises our ability to methylate which is important in our ability to detoxify, make energy, repair DNA, and deal with inflammation."[15] (More about methylation in chapter 19.)

Although volumes of research regarding the health hazards of amalgams had been documented long before Rick's health collapse, mercury had never been linked as a potential problem by his traditionally trained dentists or his conventional health practitioners. Nor was I aware of this problem; they filled my mouth too. This may have served as a contributing factor in the development of my brain tumor, which fortunately proved benign. All the consequences resulting from toxic impact are interminable.

Regarding the hazards of mercury dental amalgams, the International Academy of Oral Medicine and Toxicology (IAOMT) warns: "Mercury vapor is continuously emitted from dental amalgam fillings, and much of this mercury is absorbed and retained in the body. The output of mercury can be intensified by the number of fillings and other activities, such as chewing, teeth-grinding, and the consumption of hot liquids. Mercury is also known to be released during the placement, replacement, and removal of dental amalgam fillings."[16]

Additionally, the dentist treating Rick in the state mental hospital did not extract his abscessed teeth according to safe removal procedures established by the IAOMT. Without removing dental amalgams safely, patients are at greater risk of additional hazardous mercury exposure from the extraction.[17] From reviewing the research, Rick's mouthful of amalgams had undoubtedly exacerbated his toxic load, as evidenced by his elevated mercury levels from his multiple, heavy metals tests.

Among mercury's problematic presence in your body, mercury from dental amalgams can accumulate in the thyroid gland. The thyroid makes, stores, and releases thyroid hormones into the blood stream, controlling multiple functions. *Hashimoto's encephalopathy*, an autoimmune thyroid disease, had been listed as a possible diagnosis on Rick's discharge from Johns Hopkins in June 2004. This information was shared with all Rick's subsequent health professionals, but no one further investigated his thyroid. Again, I wonder why.

The IAOMT has chronicled (and promotes) research that dental amalgams are a source of significant mercury exposure, and a hazard to health. To learn more about biological dentistry visit their website at www.IAOMT.org.

Although it might seem obvious that dental conditions and materials can influence the entire human system, there is a clear need for the mainstream medical community, policy makers, and the public to be educated about this reality.[18]

International Academy of Medicine & Toxicology

Part 3

An Evolving Health Paradigm

—

Functional Medicine and the Biology-Based Approach to Health

Chapter 18
Conventional/Western Medicine vs. Functional/Integrative Medicine

Before the emergence and then predominance of drugs, surgical procedures, and radiation the past several decades, the American healthcare model was based primarily on natural medicine. It focused on the value of natural agents, such as food, herbs, and tissue manipulation for disease prevention and healing.

The reigning medical system in the US has since shifted to a model that is alternately termed "allopathic," "conventional," "traditional," or "Western." As science learns more about the root causes of disease, another evolving medical model, known as "functional medicine," is helping to transform patient health.

The Institute for Functional Medicine describes this medical model as "a systems biology–based approach that focuses on identifying and addressing the root cause of disease."[1] It views the body as an integrated, holistic system. This stands in contrast to conventional medicine, which views the body as a collection of different organs, with specific symptoms treated by medical specialties.

This chapter explores the distinctive differences between these two medical models.

The Conventional/Allopathic Model

The predominant medical care in the US is based on a model in which doctors and healthcare professionals treat the symptoms of disease with traditional tools of drugs, surgery, chemotherapy, radiation, and equipment. We celebrate these health professionals in their skillful and tireless handling of acute and emergency care.

Medical insurance generally covers at least a portion of patient expenses related to these providers. However, some therapies once considered alternative—such as acupuncture and chiropractic care—are increasingly covered by insurance due to their clinically proven results.

Conventional medicine shines when there is a known connection between the cause of a disease, such as setting and rehabbing a broken bone, or in the case of bacterial infections treated with antibiotics. Generally, mainstream medicine's evaluations do not usually look at the root causes, e.g., toxic exposure, chronic inflammation, diet, and other factors underlying a patient's symptoms. If conventional testing uncovers nothing obvious, then symptoms may be dismissed or attributed solely to stress or psychiatric causes.

Through Rick's 12-year illness, conventional diagnostics and therapies were not effective in treating his condition. Rick underwent a battery of tests, followed by doctors prescribing medications that masked his deeper, underlying issues. As related previously, his chronic inflammation from lifetime exposures to chemicals, heavy metals, biotoxins, and other inflammatory factors were never really addressed by his conventional medical team.

"There are both strengths and weaknesses in conventional medicine, where a specialist treats every part of your body. This style of medicinal care is called *reductionism*, i.e., neurologists for the brain, gastroenterologists for the digestive system, cardiologists for the heart, and so on.

This compartmentalization of the body system results in a more disjointed approach to addressing disease. When we create these artificial divisions, we lose sight of the body as an interconnected whole, failing to understand how different systems maybe actually related to a common, underlying cause.

Functional/integrative practitioners understand how the body must be treated as an integrative whole, to treat the specific disease or imbalance."

Dan Watts, MD

The beauty of integrative medicine is its ability to take Western, conventional medicine training with its modern understanding of the human body and modern therapeutic techniques and integrate it with ancient healing traditions and naturopathic practices. It is not simply using ancient healing philosophies to "complement" medical practice or to use them as an "alternative" to conventional medicine.[2]

Dr. Anita Sadaty

What Is The Difference Between Functional & Conventional Medicine?

Functional Medicine vs. Conventional Medicine

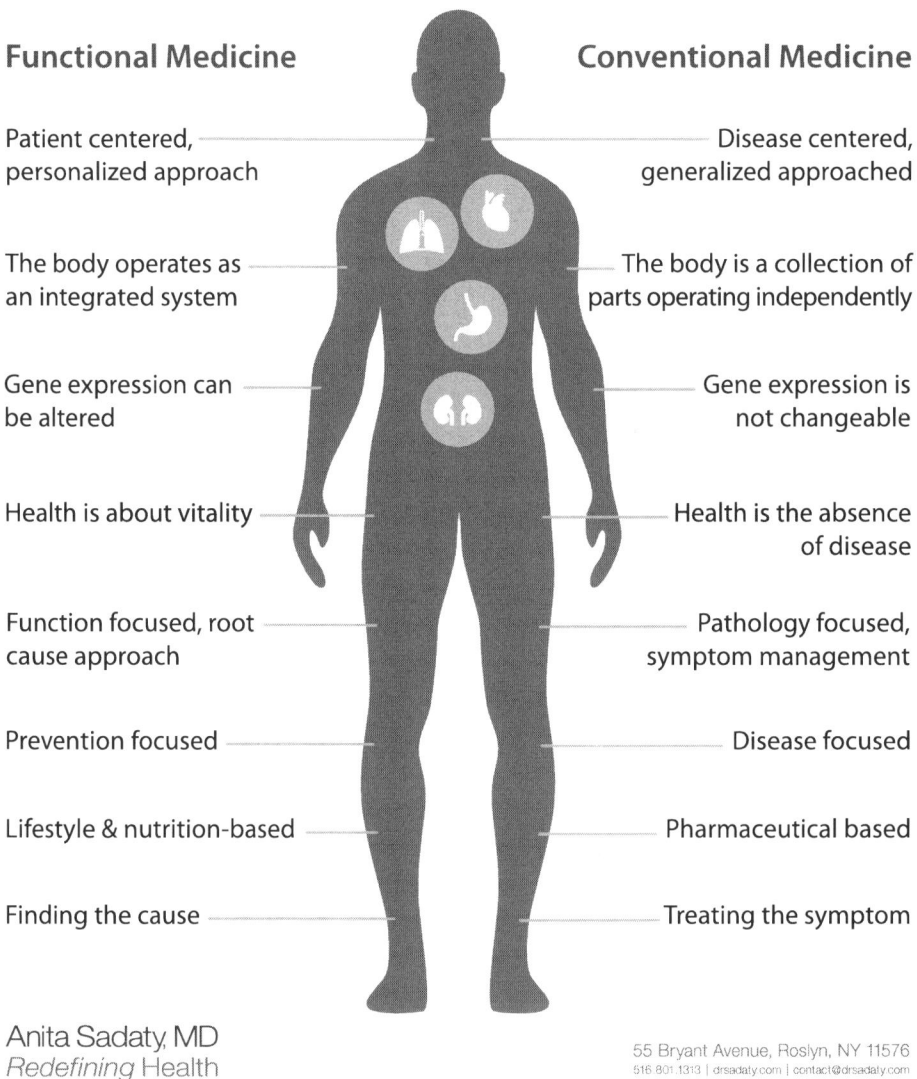

Functional Medicine	Conventional Medicine
Patient centered, personalized approach	Disease centered, generalized approached
The body operates as an integrated system	The body is a collection of parts operating independently
Gene expression can be altered	Gene expression is not changeable
Health is about vitality	Health is the absence of disease
Function focused, root cause approach	Pathology focused, symptom management
Prevention focused	Disease focused
Lifestyle & nutrition-based	Pharmaceutical based
Finding the cause	Treating the symptom

Anita Sadaty, MD
Redefining Health

55 Bryant Avenue, Roslyn, NY 11576
516 801 1313 | drsadaty.com | contact@drsadaty.com

Reprinted with permission

The Functional/Integrative Model

Fortunately, more and more doctors are choosing to practice the medical model recognized by various names: integrative, functional, holistic, or regenerative medicine. Many similarities (and some differences) are blended into their patient-centered care. These practitioners, many with medical degrees, are "root cause rebels," pursuing the causes of illnesses and offering different therapies to recover health.

Integrative medicine has been defined as "the practice of medicine that reaffirms the importance of the relationship between practitioner and patient, focuses on the whole person, is informed by evidence, and makes use of all appropriate therapeutic approaches, healthcare professionals and disciplines to achieve optimal health and healing."[3]

The functional model is based on the concept that one condition can have many causes, and conversely, that one cause can have many conditions. It identifies imbalances through specialized biomarkers to pinpoint the cause(s) of illnesses—a defining difference from conventional care for improving or restoring health. It offers individualized therapies, tailored to treat underlying causes of illness and to prevent them.

Many functional practitioners utilize "the GOTOIT framework," a system to Gather, Organize, Order, Initiate, and Track. The physician follows each patient throughout this process, assessing unhealthy patterns, finding the root cause of an issue, and creating personalized treatments and lifestyle modifications for health recovery. This strategy is important to find imbalances to prevent illnesses or to restore optimum functioning among all physiologic functions in the body.[4]

With its focus on Hippocrates' ancient proclamation, "Let thy food be thy medicine and thy medicine be thy food," functional/integrative practitioners use food, herbs, and supplements for both disease prevention and health recovery. They focus on diets rich in nutritious foods, needed supplements for nutrient diversity, and detoxification for toxic-laden bodies, and encouraging positive lifestyle choices for long-term health. Both models offer longer consultations and emphasize minimally invasive therapies, such as mind-body approaches, nutrition, prevention, and lifestyle changes.

Functional medicine practitioners conduct comprehensive genetic, environmental, nutritional, and lifestyle assessments, looking for critical clues to the underlying causes of a patient's symptoms. Using specialized diagnostics and therapies, they can identify and treat the underlying issues and help the body to heal itself, removing symptoms, not just alleviating them.

Chapter 19
Revelations from a Functional Perspective

A turning point in Rick's evaluation was our consultation with Dr. Shoemaker, the physician and passionate researcher devoted to recognizing and treating biotoxic illnesses. He evaluated Rick using precision testing of biomarkers, which identified Rick's toxic body burden as the root of his rampant inflammation and decline. Dr. Shoemaker prescribed a detoxification protocol, which dramatically improved Rick's health. He also recommended a "no-amylose diet" to further reduce inflammation. This diet forbids roots and tubers—white and sweet potatoes, beets, peanuts, and other vegetables that grow underground—and such foods as bananas, rice, oats, barley, and anything with added sugars, sucrose, corn syrup, or maltodextrin.[1]

Functional medicine uses specialized tests, e.g., toxic heavy metals analysis, mycotoxins panels, nutritional evaluations, genetic and hormone testing, and others to identify sources of inflammation and imbalances. Then practitioners use targeted therapies, including detoxification, hormone balancing, and dietary changes and supplementation to support optimum health. I saw firsthand how these perspectives made a decisive difference in evaluation and treatment.

During one of my earlier consultations with Dr. Watts, he related the experience that he and his wife, Sherry, had with mold illness and their recoveries using integrative therapies. This proved to be invaluable knowledge since I would later discover my own mold-related issues.

I have asked Dr. Watts to share his expertise regarding common tests used in functional practices and why these are useful in assessments by these practitioners.

Integrative Insights from Dr. Watts

When I went to medical school in the 1960s, we were taught how to diagnose and treat diseases through means of drugs and surgery. This model has worked well for teaching young men and women the healing arts as it is a quick and simple model. It worked well for me as I began my practice, first as an emergency room physician and later as an OB/GYN.

However, as I grew older and more experienced, questions began bubbling up:

• Are we doing all we can to help our patients?

- Why do we wait until a disease state occurs before beginning treatment?

- What about treating a disease before the disease occurs?

- What about finding the root cause of diseases?

- Why do we wait until chronic conditions, such as heart disease, cancer, cognition decline, and arthritis devastate the bodies of our patients until we are called to action?

- Are there ways to slow down, stop, reverse these chronic maladies?

The traditional model of medicine teaches little about answering these questions.

When I attended my first integrative/functional medical conference, my eyes were opened to the world of preventive and lifestyle medicine. Here, the approach was one of finding the root cause of the disease then applying lifestyle (mother nature's) tools, i.e., nutrition, supplementation, exercise, detoxification, and herbs as modalities of treatment. This root cause model requires unique lab profiles I had not previously been taught:

- Genomics/Nutrigenomics

- Organic Acids tests

- Neurotransmitters

- Hormone Balance

- Closed Chain Kinetics

- Toxic Profiles: Heavy Metals/ Biotoxins/Organotoxins

These and many other unique lab tests added many more tools to my traditional tool chest of medical care.

Since moving to Florida and having my health supervised by Dr. Watts, I am grateful for the distinctive advantage functional testing offers to patients and recognize its role in supporting wellness. Prior to my initial consultation, I provided a very detailed medical history in which I shared my former VCS screening for mycotoxins. Dr. Watts recommended repeating the VCS test, which indicated a likelihood of biotoxic exposure, which was followed up with mycotoxin testing, revealing the presence of several mold strains.

He prescribed a detoxification protocol, including supplements to enhance detoxification and recommended using an infrared sauna to help me sweat out those treacherous toxins. I was tested again a year later. Although it indicated the reduction of some strains, now a new and different one appeared. Since the results from an earlier genetics test, revealed methylation issues, I pursued further analysis.

A review of my methylation process confirmed issues, with recommendations for additional supplements. My methylation review confirms big improvements, which is reflected in my feelings of vibrant wellness.

It is with much gratitude that my health status has improved with the wisdom provided through functional testing and supervision. Now, with insights into my genetics as a poor detoxifier, and additional knowledge gained from heavy metals and biotoxin testing, I have become even more proactive with my health.

The fields of integrative and functional medicine take advantage of the power of traditional medicine, combined with the art of natural medicine.

As time goes by, more and more conventional doctors are becoming aware of the importance of the functional medicine approaches, i.e., epigenomic medicine, methylation, APOE, cancer genomics, vitamin therapy for boosting the immune system, heart health, correcting osteoporosis, and probiotics for gut health, are just a few examples. These tests can be decisive in patients' destinies.

***

Essential Evaluations

Patient evaluations through targeted testing provide the functional practitioner with a holistic perspective of a patient's health status. These include tests for:

- Inflammation
- Immune system
- Toxic exposure
  - Biotoxin screening
  - Heavy metals testing
- Nutritional evaluation
- Food sensitivity testing
- Microbiome
- Fasting insulin level
- Genetics/methylation
- Infections

- Homocysteine levels

- Hormonal status

- Blood-brain barrier

- BMI (body mass index)

- Prediabetes

Cognitive Assessment

As we age, evaluating our brain health and cognition is essential. As highlighted throughout this book, cognitive function can decline as a result of many risk factors, so early evaluation is advised to detect potential issues. Traditionally, the MMSE (Mini Mental State Exam) has long served as the standard screening tool for assessing cognitive function, yet has its limitations. While it includes tests for impairments in orientation, attention, memory, language, and visual and spatial skills, it does not identify potential risk factors for cognitive decline or the more specific nature of a brain's abnormalities.

As mentioned previously, many of Rick's medical evaluations included MMSE screenings and he scored within normal limits, leading his medical providers to rule out dementia. Although the MMSE contributes to a diagnosis of dementia, it should not be used alone to confirm or exclude a disease. What would have provided needed insights into the exact nature of his illness was still under development, soon to appear on the horizon, and revolutionary in its assessment of cognitive function and addressing potential issues.

After decades of researching neurodegeneration, Dr. Bredesen's team developed a revolutionary cognitive assessment using a series of screening tests that identified 36 contributing causes of decline. These must be holistically addressed to help prevent, as well as provide successful treatment in restoring cognitive function. Doctor Bredesen coined this comprehensive evaluation, a *cognoscopy*. In the same way a colonoscopy serves as an important periodic exam beginning at age 50 to screen for colorectal cancer, a cognoscopy evaluates the potential contributors and risk factors of cognitive decline, with recommendations to begin these assessments at age 45.

This comprehensive evaluation includes blood tests, genetic testing, specialized MRIs, and mental status exams to provide a snapshot of a patient's current cognitive abilities. These serve a dual purpose, both for prevention as well as identifying any areas requiring intervention to assist in reversing neurodegeneration. Since neurodegeneration takes many years — often decades — to develop, this provides a relatively large window of opportunity, not only to prevent but also to reverse cognitive decline through the repair and proper maintenance of these 36 potential issues.

Included as part of the cognoscopy is volumetric brain imaging, an added feature to the traditional MRI. It helps identify any regions of the brain which might be shrinking and useful in conjunction with other clinical findings as part of a patient's assessment. Generalized atrophy is more typical for Type 3 (toxic) Alzheimer's disease. When atrophy is confined to the hippocampus, other types of Alzheimer's are indicated. [2]

During the course of Rick's intensive medical evaluations, a cognoscopy with such comprehensive functional evaluation, would have offered invaluable insights. While his repeated MRIs continually indicated generalized brain atrophy, this diagnostic tool would have served a defining role. However, volumetric brain imaging was still on the horizon and now thankfully, available for securing a more in-depth analysis.

With its revolutionary application in both prevention and proven intervention regarding neurodegeneration, the cognoscopy is transforming patient prognoses and health destinies. The earlier the detection of cognitive issues, the better the chance of avoiding debilitating cognitive decline, and with opportunities for the greatest improvement. What a gift for humanity knowing this once irreversible disease no longer seals a dreaded fate!

The Miracle of Food and Nutrition

The food you eat can either be the safest and most powerful form of medicine, or the slowest form of poison.[3]

Ann Wigmore

In my career promoting wellness, I've long embraced my appreciation of nature's delicious cornucopia. With recognition of how valuable fresh fruits and vegetables are to support a healthy microbiome and body, I encourage creating menus and snacks from a rainbow of colorful fruits and vegetables. I am grateful for the growing selection or organic produce, and the previously mentioned EWG "Clean Fifteen" list for helping consumers choose safer options.

The foundation of holistic medicine recognizes the power of food and nutrition for optimum health and well-being including:

- Organic fresh fruits and vegetables

- Grass-fed meats

- Wild-caught fish, especially salmon and sardines

- Healthy fats (i.e., coconut, olive, and avocado oil)

- Non-GMO, certified organic labels on fresh and packaged foods

- Fermented foods

Research shows that allergies, immune impairment, autoimmune disease, degenerative neurological diseases, diabetes, and cancers that have become so common are not normal but are instead due to nutrient deficiencies and an ever-growing toxic load. [4]

Dr. Joseph Pizzorno

Functional medicine also recognizes how dietary imbalances can create specific health issues. For example, anxiety, depression, behavioral, and other mental health issues are often linked to a poor diet. Research reveals that our emotions are directly connected to our digestive system. As detailed previously, 95% of serotonin—the "feel good neurotransmitter"—is produced in the GI tract, not the brain. Its production is influenced by the "good" bacteria in our GI tract, and rallies against "bad" bacteria that affects mood.

Several studies have demonstrated the powerful effect of B vitamins on a wide range of neurological and psychiatric conditions and mood disorders. Brain fog and memory problems are two of the top warning signs of a vitamin B_{12} deficiency. "Symptoms of a deficiency often mimic those of dementia, such as memory loss, disorientation, and difficulty thinking and reasoning," says nutritionist Stephanie Middleberg.[5] Vitamins B_6, folate and B_{12} help regulate the synthesis and breakdown of brain chemicals, serotonin, melatonin, and dopamine involved in controlling mood. A deficiency in one or more can contribute to depression, cognitive impairment, and dementia.[6]

Folic acid and vitamins B_6 and B_{12} also impact levels of homocysteine, an amino acid found in blood plasma. High levels of homocysteine are linked to an increased risk of dementia, heart disease, stroke, and osteoporosis.[7] These vitamins impact the methylation cycle (see below) and are required for the production and proper function of neurotransmitters and the maintenance of myelin, the fatty sheath surrounding nerve cells. Without this protective coating, nerve signals become slow and sporadic, which can lead to motor function problems, cognitive losses, and changing moods.

A 2013 study revealed B vitamins slowed brain shrinkage in regions of the brain known to be most severely impacted by dementia.[8] Shrinkage was decreased by as much as 700%. By taking high doses of folic acid, vitamins B_6 and B_{12}, participants lowered their blood levels of homocysteine, a marker of inflammation, and brain shrinkage was significantly decreased by as much as 90%.[9]

(See chapter 20 "Smart Choices in Today's Toxic Times," for more detail regarding anti-inflammatory dietary recommendations.)

The Importance of Methylation Evaluations

If you have a shortage of methyl groups, or your methylation cycle is interrupted, any or all of these processes can become compromised, and you will get sick. In fact, research has clearly linked impaired methylation with all autoimmune conditions! [10]

Michelle Corey, functional mind-body practitioner and nutritionist

In all the consultations we had with Rick's specialists—neurologists, gastroenterologists, psychiatrists, internists, and others—no one addressed any impairments of his methylation cycle. Problems with these critical biochemical processes seemingly were not on the radar of conventional medical practitioners back then; I did not learn about their significance until after Rick's death. Fortunately, more practitioners are aware of the importance of epigenomic medicine, with a patient's methylation capabilities being one of the more significant in their evaluations.

Methylation plays a vital role in wellness and crucial for many processes. Efficient methylation and sulfation (AKA demethylation) cycles optimally control everything from your brain chemistry, detoxification, energy production, mood regulation, mental health, stress response and more.

As Dr. Mark Hyman states in *The UltraMind Solution*: "Problems with methylation and sulfation are involved in all mental illness and neurological dysfunction, especially depression, autism, attention deficit disorder, Alzheimer's, Parkinson's, and more. They are also responsible for heart disease and cancer." … The good news is that these processes can be almost completed fixed through diet, detoxification, and special nutritional supplements, even if you have "bad" genes."[11]

Methylation takes the nutrients from our food and supplements and uses them for energy for countless critical functions in the body:

- Genetic expression and repair of the DNA

- Inflammation response

- Detoxification of hormones, chemicals, and heavy metals

- Production and recycling of glutathione, a master antioxidant and protector of your cells

- Neurotransmitter production and synthesis affecting mood and brain chemistry

- Energy production and mitochondrial health

- Immune response to fight infections

- Reproductive functions

Genetic factors and modifiable factors can alter the epigenetic regulation of methylation pathways. Nutrition is one of the strongest modifiable factors, which plays a direct role in DNA methylation pathways.[12]

An efficient sulfation cycle is dependent on the production of glutathione, a vital antioxidant, which can only be produced effectively if both the methylation and sulfation cycles are operating well. The sulfation process helps to soak up and release toxins from the body. If the toxic load is not too great, glutathione is recycled within the body. If not, toxicity builds up in the body, creating more oxidative stress, and correspondingly, more inflammation.

The sulfur in glutathione collects the toxic waste and toxic heavy metals in the cells and sends it to the urine or stool for waste removal. When our bodies are overwhelmed from toxins, oxidative stress, or when sulfation and methylation cycles are not working well—through a lack of sulfur, or the nutrients of B_{12}, B_6 and folate—chronic health issues surface, including autoimmune illnesses.[13]

Methylation also plays a role in making and breaking down various neurotransmitters, such as energy-producing epinephrine and sleep-producing melatonin. An excess number of neurotransmitters may trigger such issues as seizures, insomnia, panic attacks, and fits of rage, all experienced by Rick following the manifestation of his long illness.

Dr. Donielle (Doni) Wilson, a naturopathic doctor, clinical nutritionist and researcher, lists some of the factors that create stress on the methylation cycle including environmental toxins, including mold, heavy metals (e.g., mercury, lead and aluminum), and inflammation due to food sensitivities and leaky gut all slow down the methylation cycle.[14]

Researchers and health professionals familiar with the methylation process have associated many conditions to methylation defects. The following list includes just some of the issues that can result from a faulty methylation cycle, which relate to many of the same conditions that Rick had been diagnosed with or we suspected he had:

- Chronic fatigue

- Dementia/Alzheimer's

- Schizophrenia

- Anxiety

- Neuropathy

- Bipolar or manic depression

- Multiple chemical sensitivities

- Insomnia

- Lyme disease[15]

The Detox Troublemaker—MTHFR, the Mutant Gene

MTHFR is a key enzyme, which if mutated, can interfere with the body's ability to perform normally in countless, critical functions. MTHFR variants are found in people worldwide with variations related to ethnicity, some having at least one MTHFR variant as high as 50%. Between 10%-15% of the Caucasian population and more than 25% of the Latino population have variants in both copies of the MTHFR gene.[16] This gene provides instructions for making an enzyme called methylenetetrahydrofolate reductase (MTHFR), which converts folate from food into l-methylfolate, necessary for methylation.

However, problems in the methylation pathway are not always genetic. If there is a deficiency of methylfolate in the body, it can create a deficiency of glutathione, leading to toxin build up in the blood and tissues. Low levels of glutathione, often referred to as "the master antioxidant," can manifest many conditions, including chronic fatigue, fibromyalgia, multiple chemical sensitivities, and neurological conditions.

If you are not able to methylate properly, you cannot produce CoQ_{10}, carnitine, creatine, or ATP (energy). You might also have nerve pain, termed "neuropathy," because the methylation process helps to make the protective wrapping around the nerves.

Some factors contributing to methylation deficiencies include:[17]

- Poor nutrition

- Stress and oxidative stress

- Medications and over-the-counter medications including antacids, acid blockers, proton pump inhibitors, corticosteroids, estrogen-containing drugs

- Gastrointestinal issues

- Inflammation

- Poor microbiome/probiotic

- Genetic traits

- Chemicals/toxins

- Heavy metals (mercury, lead, aluminum)

- Candida

- Autoimmune antibodies

- Elevated nitrous oxide from chronic inflammation, autoimmunity, Lyme disease

- Alcohol, which shuts down your methylation and depletes your glutathione stores.

Although no healthcare provider ever mentioned that Rick ever had such a test, Rick could check off almost every factor listed above! His inflammation numbers were off the charts, and testing revealed chemicals, toxins, heavy metals, pathogens, and autoimmune antibodies. Throughout his illness, Rick had chronic GI issues, for which doctors prescribed daily medications and suggested additional over-the-counter antacids.

> **Discovering my own methylation issues** Genetic testing revealed that I had the MTHFR genetic mutation, which was compromising my own methylation process. This required a supplement, methyl-cobalamin, a methylated form of vitamin B_{12}. This is recognized as essential for those with the MTHFR mutation. "Yet, it is not usually the complete solution for correcting methylation issues," says Dr. Rebecca Acosta of Natural Primary Care in Sarasota, Florida, who specializes in methylation evaluations via in-office consultations and telemedicine. "A complete methylation evaluation offers additional insights and for those with methylation issues as poor detoxifiers, this is an invaluable diagnostic tool."

> In reviewing my methylation report, she identified where specific enzymes were needed to assist in proper methylation. This test reflected that I had additional deficiencies requiring supplementation to get my methylation process performing optimally.

> During a follow-up consultation with Dr. Acosta, she reported that my methylation pathways had significantly improved. Most of the imbalances had been corrected by adding a few supplements into my daily routine and making a few dietary adjustments.

> A simple swab test used for the MTHFR and genetics profiling offered valuable insights regarding my ability to detoxify. It revealed important inadequacies in my methylation pathways, which over time likely would have posed a risk of serious health issues, had methylation not been addressed.

Now, I am especially confident that I am only taking the supplements my body really needs for optimum performance. This evaluation proved to be a critical tool reflective of the power of personalized medicine.

Detoxification—Reducing Today's Toxic Burden

Before our food, air, water, and consumer products became so toxic, our body's detoxification system (liver, kidneys, intestinal, lymphatic, skin, and respiratory systems), could handle the elimination of most toxic waste. However, with the enormous increase of environmental toxins, the body's ability to detoxify itself is now compromised, and the inflammatory nature of toxins is particularly hazardous to health. This is especially true for those who are genetically poor detoxifiers with methylation issues.

Functional practitioners are well-versed in detoxification protocols. Bruce Lourie and Rick Smith, authors of *Toxin Toxout*, an enlightened guide to living in the modern world, applaud those "[c]linicians doing detox medicine [who] are at the forefront of the health field and deserve tremendous respect for their pioneering spirit."[18]

Detoxification provides many benefits on a cellular level. Among them is the process of autophagy, the body's way of regenerating new, healthier cells through intermittent fasting and food restriction. In recent years, autophagy has been recognized in studies as a crucial defense mechanism against malignancy, infection, and neurodegenerative diseases. The process removes toxic proteins from the cells that are attributed to neurodegenerative diseases and provides energy and building blocks for cells in need of repair.[19]

It's very important to note that not every detoxification method is effective for releasing all toxins. This is because the body metabolizes different toxins in different ways using various pathways.[20] With today's growing popularity of detoxification, many options are available, and recommended to consult with an integrative practitioner for addressing your specific concerns.

The following list is limited to the detoxification procedures recommended for Rick, some which were used simultaneously:

- Intravenous chelation performed by an internist who used a combination of detoxification ingredients, including glutathione, which provides immune support and other valuable functions, including detoxifying metal and drug poisoning. This was used for heavy metal detoxification, but we later learned from research by Dr. Neil Nathan that glutathione can be counterproductive with some patients, especially mold patients.[21]

- A variety of homeopathy remedies and supplements were prescribed by functional and integrative practitioners—some specific for mycotoxins, Lyme, heavy metals, and immune and nutritional support. Additionally, chlorella, a green algae processed in tablet form, as well as cilantro, were prescribed for detoxing heavy metals and chemicals. It has a high affinity for heavy metals, but also mycotoxins, as well as other toxins including volatile organic compounds (VOCs), pesticides, and herbicides. Since it binds only to toxic metals, not essential minerals, it can be used long-term with no risk over time of nutritional deficiency.[22]

- Acupuncture and acupressure treatments were provided by several integrative practitioners. These treatments typically help to increase the flow of energy throughout the body, remove blockages and allow the liver to function properly, assisting the body to detox more effectively.

- Cholestyramine (Questran) treatments were started in January 2005, as prescribed by Dr. Shoemaker's protocol for CIRS. Cholestyramine binds toxins in the intestines so they can be released through the colon.

- Later, Rick was prescribed Welchol for the same purpose, which in addition to cholesterol, binds to other fat-soluble molecules and to mycotoxins. He remained on Welchol until I was legally unable to supervise his care. Since Rick's cholesterol levels were quite low, his doctors saw no need for the medication, either not recognizing or disregarding its importance and striking it from his medication orders.

- After learning about the importance of detoxification in 2005, Rick's daily routine also included an aloe-vera based mineral drink containing a variety of bioactive herbs and botanicals to bind toxins and aid in their release. These detoxifying herbs included a blend of turmeric, ashwagandha, burdock root, peppermint leaf, pau d'arco, licorice root, yellow dock, and others. The polysaccharides in the inner heart of aloe are helpful for detoxification and immune support, and encourage the liver's biochemical, toxin-neutralizing processes. These are natural "toxin hunters" which help to break apart toxins making them water soluble and able to be released.[23]

This herbal cleanse became part of Rick's daily protocol, but only while I was able to manage his care. However, while he resided for long stretches of time at hospitals and a few nursing facilities, they either refused to authorize the detoxification procedures I requested or did not administer them on a routine basis. His condition always notably declined.

The protocol for biotoxin detoxification is not standard practices in conventional medicine, yet essential for healing from sustained inflammation caused by them. A few doctors whose practices are devoted to treating biotoxic patients have successfully created alternative detoxification therapies. More advancements in laboratory testing are now able to identify specific strains of mold with specific therapies for detoxifying them.

(For additional detoxification methods, see chapter 20, "Smart Choices in Today's Toxic Times.")

On the Brink of a Paradigm Shift in Healthcare

Fortunately, an increasing number of health practitioners are embracing the functional approach for evaluating and treating patients. You can also find informative documentaries featuring functional practitioners and therapies for treating depression, anxiety, dementia, cancer, autoimmune disorders, and other conditions generally considered irreversible.

Increasingly, patients who have struggled with chronic health issues without finding relief within conventional practices are turning to functional or integrative medicine. Answers can be found there now with even more anticipated opportunities for pinpointing issues and correcting them.

Soon we'll be unraveling the fundamental basis for all these inflammatory immune responses by showing the differential gene activation - and suppression - that'll show us the genomic basis for immune responses gone wild. Soon we'll be able to provide targeted gene therapy for those who have become ill and possibly, targeted gene therapy for those at risk. Surely, the funding for this research will come.

It may seem like a simple idea, but once we know which genes are bad actors, then we should target our therapies to "shutting off" the noise made by these genes.[24]

Ritchie Shoemaker, MD

Through my consultation with functional practitioners and by following their recommendations, my lab tests are now mostly within desirable ranges. I attribute that to the wisdom revealed through functional medicine and by making health a priority. I have changed many habits, conscious of the known risks associated with inflammation. With knowledge of critical underlying causes that can ignite inflammatory conditions, I am confident my health is continually being evaluated and monitored from a functional perspective, with any potential issues addressed and averted.

If you are in the grips of a mysterious malady, walking alongside someone with one, or want to minimize your risk of developing a chronic condition for your health's sake, act now! Seek the wisdom of a functional practitioner, equipped with diagnostic tools and a proven roadmap for experiencing a different health destiny in our changing world.

Functional medicine is shifting the current health paradigm, but there is still much that needs to change. Doctors concede it often takes an average of two decades for scientific discoveries to be accepted into conventional treatment. That is too long to wait because today's troubling statistics serve as evidence that we cannot continue with the status quo, as highlighted in chapter 21, "A Wake Up Call for Us All."

While our politicians and healthcare industry leaders ponder the economics and systems for distributing healthcare, a quiet revolution is happening outside their system, and your good health will be the most important benefits. It's a welcome change, a paradigm shifting change of seismic proportions, and one that has me more excited than ever to practice the art of medicine and healing.[25]

Scott Rollins, MD

Part 4

Taking Action in Our
Inflammatory Times

Chapter 20
Smart Choices in Today's Toxic Times

The epidemics (barely acknowledged by conventional medicine) of chronic fatigue syndrome, fibromyalgia, autism, dementia, autoimmune illness, cancer, mold toxicity, and Lyme disease all share a common theme: inflammation created by an immune system that has been overstimulated and does not know how to correct itself.[1]

Neil Nathan, MD

With inflammation now known as the ignition factor for neurological issues, cancer, heart disease, diabetes, arthritis, depression, and other chronic illnesses, what can you do to reduce your risk of such a fate? Science continues to document how the power of personal habits and lifestyle choices are directly connected to reducing the body's inflammatory responses. The question each of us must answer is, "Am I willing to make necessary changes that can help minimize inflammation in my body in order to support my health?"

Often, we need a "why" to spur us into action. My "why" stemmed from witnessing Rick's health collapse, as well as the chronic, debilitating illnesses of both my parents. My father endured decades of pain and misery with heart disease, and then became extremely incapacitated with Parkinson's disease the last twelve years of his life. My mother suffered from autoimmune conditions and cancer and died from Alzheimer's. All of them experienced tragic debilitation, as was the same fate of others in our respective families.

In seeking insights regarding Rick's health issues, it became clear I needed to take action to reduce my own risks for going down the inflammatory highway. Scanning documents from the Alzheimer's Association offers plenty of reinforcement:

> "Alzheimer's disease is thought to begin 20 years or more before symptoms arise, with changes in the brain that are unnoticeable to the person affected. Only after years of brain changes do individuals experience noticeable symptoms such as memory loss and language problems. Symptoms occur because nerve cells (neurons) in parts of the brain involved in thinking, learning and memory (cognitive function) have been damaged or destroyed."[2]

The knowledge of my personal genetics, coupled with awareness of the ways I could reduce my own inflammation risks, gave me a steadfast desire to adopt the strategies to do so. Unlike other risk factors for cognitive decline that you cannot change, such as age and genetics, you *can* control diet, exercise, and other lifestyle choices. By following the collective wisdom gleaned from science, you can enhance your health by making smart choices and adopting lifestyle habits to reduce inflammation and the risks for neurological issues and other chronic conditions.

Toxin-Taming Tactics

In previous chapters, I discussed the increasing importance of detoxification due to mounting exposure to biotoxins, synthetic chemicals, heavy metals, parasites, and other pollutants that contribute to inflammation. While your body is miraculously designed to naturally detoxify, it is also under tremendous pressure due to excessive toxic overload. Therefore, supporting your body's detoxification system is very advantageous to proper functioning.

Different detoxification methods address different toxins and vary in effectiveness, so it's important to consult with a knowledgeable practitioner regarding the most efficient detoxification practices specific to your needs.

The following are some of the options available for releasing toxins to optimize your body's natural detoxification system.

- **Chelation:** See details listed in "Chelation Treatments for Heavy Metals" section in chapter 17.

- **Detox diets:** Ocean Robbins states, "If you want to detoxify, the first thing to do is to stop bringing toxins into your body in the first place. And the place to start is with the food on your plate."[3]

  Science has explored how specific foods can help your body boost its detoxifying power. Some of these include onions, garlic, cruciferous vegetables, leafy greens, apples, beets, blueberries, avocadoes, lemons, ginger, turmeric, cilantro, chlorella (a type of algae), and green tea. All are beneficial to support this vital process with their natural detoxifying powers.[4]

- **Fasting and intermittent fasting** is currently one of the most popular health and fitness trends, and for a good reason. Fasting offers a wide range of benefits regarding weight loss, metabolism, insulin resistance, lowering blood pressure and cholesterol, and reducing the potential for neurodegenerative effects.[5] Cells respond to intermittent fasting, which leads to greater antioxidant defenses, DNA repair, supporting mitochondrial function, autophagy (cleaning out damaged cells and regenerating newer, healthier cells), and the corresponding reduction of inflammation.[6] It's an eating pattern that cycles between eating and fasting.

Common intermittent fasting methods involve daily 16-hour fasts or fasting for 24 hours, twice per week. Intermittent fasting can be achieved through several methods. These are just a few:[7]

- **The 16/8 method:** This involves skipping breakfast and restricting your daily eating period to 8 hours, such as 10:00 a.m. to 6:00 p.m. Then you fast for 16 hours in between.

- **Eat-Fast-Eat:** This involves fasting for 24 hours, once or twice a week; for example, not eating from dinner on the first day until dinner the next day.

- **The 5:2 diet:** On two consecutive days of the week, you consume only 500–600 calories, but eat normally the other 5 days.

- **Infrared saunas**: Since the skin is the body's largest organ for elimination, sauna therapy enhances detoxification by inducing sweating and increasing blood flow. The deep penetration of infrared heat releases toxins from the organs to the fat tissue under the skin, then eliminated in sweat. Saunas help the liver break down and eliminate toxic chemicals and heavy metals; help lower cortisol, a core contributor to inflammation; and assist in cell regeneration, including the production of white blood cells for immune support.[8]

  Researchers have analyzed the sweat produced in both traditional and infrared saunas. From traditional saunas, the sweat was predominantly 97% water and 3% toxins. In contrast, the sweat from infrared saunas was 80-85% water, with 15-20% consisting of heavy metals, sulfuric acid, sodium, ammonia, uric acid, and other fat-soluble toxins.[9]

- **Light therapy:** used to reduce inflammation and stimulate cell regeneration, including brain cell growth.[10] (For more details about light therapy, see chapter 22.)

- **Ozone therapy**: heavily studied for more than a century, has proven to be a safe detox therapy with minimal and preventable side effects. It can be delivered through several methods, helping to inactivate bacteria, viruses, fungi, yeast, and protozoa; stimulate oxygen metabolism; and activate the immune system.[11]

- **Activated charcoal**: a carbon material made from coconut shells, wood, or other materials available in powder or capsule form, is used to bind and eliminate toxic substances in the body.[12]

- **Zeolite and bentonite clays:** are more selective than activated charcoal for binding toxins but can still bind to nutrients. They are used for binding to biotoxins from mold and other microbes but can bind to other toxins as well.[13]

- **Craniosacral therapy:** offers techniques that focus on enhancing and restoring the movement of cerebrospinal fluid within the brain and spinal cord. This facilitates proper flushing of accumulated waste products in the brain, serving as a detoxification for the brain as well as the whole body. (More about the science of this therapy in chapter 22, "An Evolving Renaissance in Brain Wellness.")

- **Optimize your methylation (detoxification) process** for its importance for proper functioning as described in chapter 19.

Nurture Your Microbiome

Changes in the gut microbiome as people age have been linked to disruptions in the immune system, persistent inflammation, and chronic diseases, including neurological disorders such as Alzheimer's.[14]

National Institute on Aging

More is being learned about the relationship between gut microbes—those tiny 100 trillion organisms in the digestive system—and aging-related processes that lead to dementia. As outlined in chapter 16, "Gut Issues—Ground Zero for Inflammation," the way these gut microbes communicate with the central nervous system influences your overall health, your brain, mood, and behavior.[15] Researchers are exploring how these changes are related to each other and to brain changes regarding neurodegeneration and the accumulation of the toxic proteins, beta-amyloid and tau, which are associated with Alzheimer's disease.

Think of your microbiome as your inner garden composed of trillions of microbes—the richer and more diverse the community, the lower your risk of disease and imbalances. With the composition of your microbiome having such a powerful influence on your brain's health, cultivating a healthy balance of microbes is in your hands, and can significantly impact your health now and in the future.

Choose a Diet to Suit Your Health Goals

Since your dietary choices are powerful building blocks to wellness, you play a critical role in directing your health destiny. You may have very specific health goals such as weight loss; meal planning with a need to accommodate food restrictions, sensitivities, or preferences; as part of a health prevention plan; to assist in healing a health condition; or simply a renewed desire to support your health to look and feel your best now, as well as reduce your risk of future issues.

Many studies regarding two different lifestyle diets, the Mediterranean and the ketogenic diet, have validated their abilities to support and transform health. By including intermittent fasting, the benefits are further magnified, providing a valuable method to achieve wellness goals.

Consider the Ketogenic Connection

The ketogenic diet, with its focus of cutting carbs and eating more fat, has gained favor especially with those seeking weight loss and metabolic health. It has many known benefits, among them as a therapeutic strategy for diabetes, cancer, cardiovascular health, and neurodegenerative support. Its primary purpose is to drop blood sugar so low that the body uses fat instead for its energy supply.[16]

With so many people now loading up on sodas, refined sugars, and refined carbohydrates as part of today's highly processed diets, they're burning sugar for energy. However, the body is designed to run more efficiently on fats than sugar to support normal metabolic signaling and cellular health. By reducing tissue damage from free radicals that cause chaos with our DNA and mitochondria, the ketogenic diet offers many proven benefits:

- Reduced inflammation
- Improved fat burning
- Mental clarity and sharpness
- Abundant energy
- Clear skin
- Reduced cravings
- Mitochondrial biogenesis*
- Anti-aging effect
- Reduced risk of chronic disease

Source: DrJockers.com, "9 Proven Benefits of a Ketogenic Diet"

*The body's capacity to produce more energy by increasing the number of mitochondria.

With the ketogenic diet, fat is your friend. The substitution of fat for carbs encourages the body to burn fat over carbs/glucose which induces ketosis, the metabolic state when your body burns fat for energy instead of blood sugar. When insulin levels are low, without enough sugar or glucose to supply the body's need for fuel, ketones are formed. These burn fat more efficiently than sugar, causing far less oxidative stress.

Diets that are high in sugar and grains place demands upon your blood glucose levels. Over time, your insulin receptors require more and more insulin to be effective, causing insulin resistance. It's estimated insulin resistance currently affects about 45% of Americans in various degrees which can lead to prediabetes, diabetes, dementia, and other issues. The ketogenic diet keeps both your blood glucose and your insulin levels low which gives your insulin receptors an opportunity to return to more efficient functioning.[17]

A pattern of blood sugar imbalance is highly damaging to the brain. When brain cells become insulin resistant, needed energy is compromised, and inflammation often results in cognitive issues. With the brain so reliant on healthy mitochondria for proper functioning, it is the first to suffer consequences of excessive oxidative stress.

Studies have shown that ketone metabolism creates lower levels of oxidative stress in comparison to glucose metabolism, effectively lowering inflammation and supporting mitochondrial health and improved levels of various neurotransmitters involved in health and disease processes. With a ketogenic diet, ketones do not require insulin to enter the cell, and can cross the blood brain barrier that separates the brain from circulation; most brain cells are able to metabolize ketones.[18]

BDNF (brain-derived neurotrophic factor) supports brain cells and regulates the growth of neural connections in the brain. Low levels of BDNF have been correlated with dementia, mental disorders, and Huntington's disease, an inherited disease that causes the progressive degeneration of nerve cells in the brain. Research has demonstrated that fasting and the ketogenic diet improve neurodegenerative disorders by making cells more responsive to BDNF. This helps to combat neurodegeneration by supporting the continued growth and development of neuronal connections. [19]

A Dynamic Duo

Combining the keto diet with intermittent fasting offers many benefits of weight loss, reduction of blood sugar and insulin levels, and the treatment and prevention of neurodegenerative conditions. Ketones and intermittent fasting both train the body to efficiently burn fat by depleting glucose and lowering insulin levels. Intermittent fasting helps to achieve higher ketone levels. Fasting, exercise, and a ketogenic diet all serve in producing ketones from body fat.

Ketones can also be generated from food sources used as supplements to stimulate or maintain ketosis, such as coconut or MCT oils (medium chain triglycerides). Neither of these contain ketones but are converted into them when following a low-carb, high-fat diet. This offers an option to support those unable to commit to either a ketogenic diet or intermittent fasting.

However, this dietary lifestyle has compelling advantages for brain health. Your body becomes efficient at burning fat and turns fat into ketones in the liver which can supply energy for the brain. The presence of ketone bodies has a neuroprotective impact on aging brain cells. It helps to reduce amyloid and tau, associated with Alzheimer's. For all these benefits, it has gained interest as a potential therapy for neurodegenerative disorders.[20] Continuing clinical trials with patients who are diagnosed with cognitive issues have demonstrated improved brain function with the ketogenic diet and intermittent fasting included in treatment protocols.[21]

Explore the Mediterranean Diet

Numerous studies have demonstrated many health benefits associated with the Mediterranean diet in helping with weight loss as well as reducing the risk of heart attacks, strokes, Type 2 diabetes, and cognitive decline. The diet is composed of fruits, vegetables, whole grains, legumes, fish, and other seafood, as well as unsaturated fats, such as olive oil. There is a corresponding reduction in the consumption of red meat, eggs, and sweets, which is associated with reducing the risk of dementia.

Researchers believe this diet might increase specific nutrients that serve to protect the brain by their anti-inflammatory and antioxidant properties. Diets that are rich in antioxidants can help your body fight oxidative stress caused by excess free radicals and other toxins that increase your risk of disease. Antioxidants may also inhibit beta-amyloid deposits, which are found in the brains of people with Alzheimer's or improve cellular metabolism in ways that protect against the disease.[22]

A variation of this diet is called MIND (Mediterranean–DASH Intervention for Neurodegenerative Delay) that incorporates the DASH (Dietary Approaches to Stop Hypertension) diet. This diet also helps to reduce high blood pressure, another risk factor associated with Alzheimer's disease.[23]

The Mediterranean diet and its variations are anti-inflammatory in nature. What you eat and drink contributes greatly to controlling or reversing inflammation.

Reduce Inflammation

> *"One of the most powerful tools to combat inflammation comes not from the pharmacy, but from the grocery store.*[24]
>
> Dr. Frank Hu, professor of nutrition and epidemiology,
> Harvard School of Public Health

Eating a varied diet of colorful plant foods has many health-enhancing benefits that go beyond the power of vitamins and minerals. Fruits and vegetables are rich sources of many nutrients that contribute to their color, taste, and smell, including a diverse group of phytonutrients—compounds also found in whole grains, nuts, seeds, and legumes.

Scientists estimate there are more than 6,000 phytonutrients (also known as phytochemicals); they are just beginning to understand their positive impact on health.[25] Phytonutrients are powerful antioxidants with anti-inflammatory and immune system benefits. Fruits, nuts, cocoa, vegetables, spices, and green tea have some of the highest amounts of antioxidants. These protect your body from damage caused by free radicals that can lead to oxidative stress, which is linked to many chronic diseases, such as cancer, diabetes, heart disease and dementia.

For example, diets rich in the polyphenol, flavonoid, are associated with the prevention of neurodegenerative and cardiovascular diseases and cancer. Quercetin in apples, onions, and citrus fruits may lower inflammation and blood pressure. Studies have linked flavonoids in berries, apples, citrus, onions, soybeans, and coffee to reduction in inflammation and tumor growth. Carotenoids in red, orange, yellow, and green plants may boost immunity and inhibit cancer growth and cardiovascular disease. Designing a diet from a rainbow of fruits and vegetables can support your health and reduce your risk of disease.[26]

Enjoy Wholesome, Anti-inflammatory Foods

> *Anything that affects the gut, always affects the brain.*[27]
> Dr. Charles Major, Harvard University

As a rule, select organic, non-GMO foods to prevent or minimize inflammation. Some of the top anti-inflammatory foods are listed here.

- **Leafy greens** are rich sources of many important vitamins and minerals including inflammatory fighting magnesium. There is considerable evidence that people with high inflammatory markers often have low magnesium levels, according to Forrest H. Nielsen, a research nutritionist at the USDA's Grand Forks Human Nutrition Research Center in North Dakota.

- **Nuts** are rich sources of nutrients, including magnesium and phytonutrients. Magnesium deficiency has been linked to insulin resistance, type 2 diabetes, hypertension, and other conditions with a common background of chronic inflammation.[28]

- **Red, purple, and blue fruits and vegetables** such as berries, grapes, cherries, and red cabbage contain anthocyanin, which gives them their vibrant coloring. These foods also contain potent antioxidants that are anti-inflammatory and support the immune system. Resveratrol, another polyphenol found in grapes and berries, has been linked to reduced risk of dementia, heart disease, cancer, and other chronic conditions.[29]

- **Fatty fish** (e.g., salmon, tuna, mackerel, sardines) serve as great sources of protein and omega-3 fatty acids, EPA and DHA. Studies have demonstrated that EPA and DHA reduce inflammation associated with chronic illnesses including metabolic syndrome, heart disease, diabetes, and kidney disease.[30] Limit varieties like tuna and mackerel, known to be higher in mercury, to no more than once weekly.

- **Cruciferous vegetables** are a diverse family of inflammatory fighters with many relatives—broccoli, cabbage, cauliflower, brussels sprouts, kale, bok choy, arugula, turnip and mustard greens, and other nutrient dense vegetables. The phytochemical, sulforaphane, fights inflammation by reducing levels of cytokines and is linked to a reduction in cancer and other chronic illnesses.[31]

- **Extra virgin olive oil,** a staple of the Mediterranean diet, provides more anti-inflammatory benefits than those of other refined olive oils. Research shows that oleocanthal, an antioxidant found in virgin olive oil, has similar anti-inflammatory benefits to ibuprofen.[32]

- **Dark chocolate and cocoa products** contain flavanols that are heralded as antioxidants, anticarcinogens, cardio-preventives, antimicrobials, and antivirals. These have neuro-protective benefits associated with a decreased risk of dementia.

The study "Flavonoids: Modulators of Brain Function?" states: "Dietary phytochemicals, in particular flavonoids, may exert beneficial effects on the central nervous system by protecting neurons against stress-induced injury, by suppressing neuroinflammation and by improving cognitive function."[33] To reap its anti-inflammatory benefits, choose dark chocolate containing at least 70% cocoa or greater.

- **Tomatoes** are high in vitamin C and an especially good source of lycopene, an antioxidant beneficial for its capacity to protect against diseases that are associated with oxidative stress and inflammation.[34]

- **Green tea** contains a unique and potent type of catechin (another inflammatory fighter) called epigallocatechin gallate (EGCG). While green tea is recognized for this polyphenol, it is also found in other teas, fruits, and vegetables, and some nuts.[35]

- **Herbs and spices** add their piquant flavoring to many foods and are also valued for their anti-inflammatory and antioxidant benefits. Among this aromatic family noted for their outstanding healthful benefits, a few include:
  - Turmeric: With its active polyphenol compound, curcumin, studies have shown its value in reducing symptoms of depression and Alzheimer's disease.[36]
  - Cinnamon: This spice has been shown to help with neurological disorders as well as exhibiting antioxidant, antidiabetic, antimicrobial, anticancer, and lipid-lowering properties.[37]
  - Ginger: As an herbal medicinal product, this spice shares pharmacological properties with non-steroidal, anti-inflammatory drugs to treat pain and inflammation. Research has shown it can limit the production of inflammatory cytokines and the activity of enzymes that promote inflammation.[38]

Supplements—giving your body what it needs

After decades of following a healthy diet, I was surprised to learn of a few deficits revealed from a nutritional evaluation via a blood test, along with some other biomarkers, signaling inflammation. I was prescribed specific supplements to support my nutritional needs and lower inflammation.

Knowing the difference these have made in my overall health and in reducing my risk of inflammation, I now think of supplements as an insurance policy to provide critical nutrients specific to my genetics and nutritional needs.

As described earlier, the era of agrichemicals has degraded the quality of our soil, and even many of today's organic foods no longer contain their once-rich nutritional content. Although a healthy diet may supply adequate nutrition, that is not the same as being sufficient in providing your body with all needed nutrients for optimum performance or keeping inflammation in check.

American consumers recognize their value. According to the Center for Responsible Nutrition's "CRN 2020 Survey on Dietary Supplements," nearly three-quarters of Americans report taking dietary supplements and more than 80% of adults 55+ in the US take dietary supplements. Overall health/wellness benefits were cited by 40% of the respondents for taking dietary supplements and 32% consume supplements to support their immune health. The third reason: to fill nutrient gaps in their diet for energy.

"Results from the 2020 survey continue to demonstrate an intensified focus on ingredients to support overall health and wellness and immunity," says CRN's Brian Wommack, senior vice president, communications.[39]

Limit Consumption of Inflammatory Foods and Beverages

- Refined carbohydrates: white bread, pasta, white rice, crackers, flour tortillas, biscuits, pastries

- Fast food, convenience meals

- Sugary or salty snack foods

- Fried foods: Fried chicken, French fries, egg rolls, doughnuts

- Sugar or artificially sweetened beverages: soda, sweet tea, and sports and energy drinks

- Red meat

- Processed meats: bacon, deli meats, hot dogs, sausages

- Trans fats: shortening, partially hydrogenated vegetable oil, margarine

- Alcohol

- Eliminate artificial sweeteners: Switch to organic stevia, a natural sweetener

More Microbiome-Loving Strategies

Eat fermented foods: Probiotics are vital to protect the complex gut-brain-immune system and supply a rich diversity for a healthy microbiota. They contain live microorganisms which are powerful for both the body and brain, improve digestion, support detoxification, reduce depression, and support heart health. If these beneficial microbes are not replenished, your immune system can be compromised.

Probiotics are found in fresh, fermented vegetables, such as sauerkraut, pickles, miso, and kimchi; in fermented dairy products such as yogurt and kefir; and kombucha, a sparkling, slightly sweet beverage filled with beneficial bacteria, amino acids, B vitamins and enzymes. They contain live microorganisms which are valuable for health—improving digestion, reducing depression, and supporting heart health.

Take a probiotic supplement: Effective probiotic supplements support colonization of the intestinal tract, crowding out disease-causing bacteria, yeasts, and viruses. Probiotics not only improve gut health, but research shows they may also enhance cognitive function and mood as well as lowering stress and anxiety.[40]

Consider taking digestive enzymes: Enzymes are the catalysts for every biochemical process that takes place inside your body. Digestive enzymes are found in raw and living food and help to pre-digest food, extract the nutrients, and deliver them throughout the body. Yet, heat from food processing, pasteurization, and cooking, destroys them, rendering them unable to perform the vital functions of digestion and the assimilation of nutrients.

With changes to our food supply, including over-processing and nutritional deficiencies, many of us lack the enzymes we need for optimal health. Without necessary natural enzymes, the body must produce extra enzymes to digest food and extract nutrients, which puts more strain on vital GI organs like the pancreas. When diminished enzyme production becomes chronic, it results in poor digestion and compromises the body's ability to eliminate toxins, repair cell tissue, and perform other vital functions.

Fill up on fiber: Dietary fiber is a crucial component of a healthy diet and an important player when it comes to the gut microbiome. A high-fiber diet has been studied for its ability to lower inflammation by modifying both the pH and the permeability of the gut.[41] Soluble fiber found in fruits, vegetables, grains, beans, and seeds is considered prebiotic. It is broken down by the gut bacteria, providing diversity and stimulating the growth of healthy bacteria. A subtype of soluble fiber, inulin, is found in chicory root, onions, garlic, leeks, bananas, Jerusalem artichokes, asparagus, oats, apples, and flax.[42]

Take antibiotics only when necessary: A single course of antibiotics can change the composition of oral and gut microbiomes for at least a year, according to a modelling study by researchers at University College London. This leads to a decrease in the number and types of microbes found in the gut, impacting beneficial diversity.[43]

Monitor your emotions and manage stress: With the gut-brain axis now recognized as the "second brain," the gut is indeed extremely sensitive to emotions. Fear, anger, anxiety, sadness, and other negative states churn up both the microbiome and biochemical actions within the brain. Taking charge of your emotions is vital for managing mood and for minding a healthy microbiome.

Repeated stress is a major trigger for persistent inflammation, putting both your physical and mental health at risk, with enormous impact on your brain. When stress becomes chronic, the blood-brain barrier becomes leaky, circulating inflammatory proteins into the brain.[44]

Prolonged levels of cortisol, the stress hormone, is linked to mood disorders as well as shrinkage of the hippocampus. Especially vulnerable to such insults, the hippocampus is a critical brain region for learning and memory. Inflammation can also adversely affect brain systems linked to motivation and mental agility.[45]

With awareness of the wide-ranging impact of stress upon the body, I have found mastering stress reduction habits to be the most challenging—monitoring situations that invoke responses of worry, conflict, irritation, or otherwise yank me from my desired state of well-being.

As the coauthor of *Get Along with Anyone,* I have presented many stress-reduction workshops and shared strategies for setting desired intentions and choosing thoughts, feelings, and actions to shift to more elevated states of well-being. To be honest, I still have times where it is challenging to handle stressful situations with grace and ease! I have encountered plenty of "tests" along life's path to respond in accordance with my best intentions. However, knowing that inner peace is both my desire and personal responsibility, I must consciously rise above the clamor to support my intention and respond accordingly. Otherwise, I just ramp up unwanted cortisol, my immune system takes a hit, and I experience the consequences of not acting in harmony with my desires.

I rely on a few techniques when facing stress-inducing situations:

1. Review what is within your control and take needed actions.

2. Use time-tested breathwork and stress-reducing tools.

3. Develop a practice of mindfulness, bringing awareness to the present moment, and reflection into your day. A growing body of evidence documents the power of meditation for a wide variety of benefits. This is true not only for stress reduction, but for broad support for mental, emotional, and physical well-being. Research suggests that a wide range of symptoms or conditions can be improved including anxiety, chronic pain, cancer, depression, heart disease, irritable bowel syndrome and many others—all compelling reasons for taking time for a mental R and R.[46]

I share more about my experiences in dealing with my own fear, worry, anxiety, and stress as a caregiver in Part 5, "Strategies for Managing Life's Uncertainties."

Beyond Minding Your Microbiome

Exercise

Low grade chronic inflammation is associated with both the aging process and chronic medical conditions. Exercise is valuable for all ages as both a preventative measure and for reducing inflammation.

Regarding brain health, it increases neurogenesis—the production of new brain cells—for your mood, cognition, and physical health. As reported in a *Wall Street Journal* article, "What Science Tells Us about Preventing Dementia," a 6-month study of sedentary seniors with mild memory issues, showed a significant reduction in the level of tau protein, which accumulates in the brains of people with Alzheimer's, from levels in their spinal fluid.[47]

There is good news for all who are exercise challenged! As reported in the journal, *Brain, Behavior and Immunity,* research reveals that exercise does not have to be rigorous to gain anti-inflammatory benefits. Twenty minutes of moderate exercise, which includes brisk walking, appears to be sufficient. Strenuous workouts for a long duration are not required, but daily exercise provides powerful, anti-inflammatory support.[48]

The American Heart Association recommends 150 minutes of moderate-intensity aerobic activity or 75 minutes per week of vigorous aerobic activity, or a combination ideally spread throughout the week.[49]

Manage Weight Wellness

Those who are overweight or obese have higher rates of inflammation with a corresponding higher risk for many of the diseases associated with it. Mid-life obesity increases the risk of developing late-life Alzheimer's disease. With obesity's influence early in the development of neurological issues, achieving weight wellness is a critical consideration.[50]

Get Sufficient Sleep

If you have trouble getting to sleep or staying asleep, here are some tips which are helpful for achieving quality sleep.

- Aim for 7 to 9 hours of sleep nightly. Set a schedule to go to bed and wake up at the same time each day.

- Exercise daily but no later than a few hours before going to bed.

- Create a relaxing environment for sleeping. Try aromatherapy with essential oils. Research studies have demonstrated their positive benefits upon sleep.[51] Lavender, vanilla, rose, jasmine, citrus, and other essential oils diffused into the sleeping environment support sleep, stress, and pain relief, and help to regulate mood.[52]

- Avoid bright lights, loud sounds, and keep the room at a comfortable temperature. Turn off all screen devices at least an hour prior to bedtime.

- Take time to relax before going to bed, perhaps including a cup of herbal tea. Chamomile, valerian root, and lavender teas are regarded as natural sleep enhancers. Avoid caffeine and nicotine products late in the day and alcohol before bed.

- If you cannot get to sleep, get up, read, listen to calming music, or other relaxing activity until you feel tired.

- Consult with your health practitioner if you continue having sleep issues. Most sleep disorders can be treated effectively.[53]

Enjoy Healthy Social Connections

Research shows the many benefits of maintaining social connectedness for physical, mental, and emotional wellness. Our connections with friends and family are part of a flourishing life and work wonders for our well-being when challenges arise. Studies show that positive social connections can lower inflammation, support the immune system, and increase longevity by as much as 50%! Not surprisingly, one study showed that lack of social connection is a greater detriment to health than obesity, smoking, and high blood pressure.[54]

As an extrovert social connectedness comes rather easily to me, knowing it's a priority for maintaining my personal well-being. The current COVID-19 restrictions and "social distancing" thwart vital mixing and mingling of hearts and souls for humanity's highest expression.

Never underestimate the power of connection—for a healthy life, eat right, exercise and connect!

Strategies for Tackling Toxic Exposures

In chapter 14, I spotlighted the pervasive nature of toxins in our daily lives. Although we cannot avoid toxins altogether, we can be diligent in reducing our risks of exposure.

Air Purifiers

Air purifiers help to reduce the amount of harmful microparticles, such as mold spores, allergens, viruses, and other contaminants by drawing air through a filter, removing the impurities, and releasing clean air back into the indoor environment.

Mold releases spores into the air, contributing to increased toxic exposure and causing inflammatory responses especially in mold-sensitive people. Breathing clean, fresh air is especially important if you have mold sensitivities; however, the respiratory systems of those without mold-specific allergies can also be irritated and inflamed wherever the air is laden with greater concentrations of mold spores.[55]

Indoor mold grows in the presence of water, such as seepage from foundation walls, basement floors, or defective plumbing. Mold can be visible on surfaces or lurking behind drywall, shower tiles, in attics, under carpets, or any damp environment.

The High Efficiency Particulate Air (HEPA) filter is generally most effective for removing airborne mold spores. The HEPA standard is based on the ability to remove 99.97% of particles that are 0.3 microns in size or greater.[56] If there is an area in your house where mold is or might be an issue—like a poorly ventilated bathroom, kitchen, or basement—an air purifier is critical for removing mold spores and reducing their spread. The HEPA filter traps and kills airborne mold spores before they reproduce, making it a wise investment for ensuring indoor air quality.

Mold Inspection and Remediation

A professional mold inspection can assist in evaluating whether your living environment is free of hazardous mold. This is especially advised if you are experiencing a range of symptoms associated with toxicity. As described in our story, both Rick and I had decades of exposure to mold, yet conventional medicine had not yet linked it to serious health issues.

Ironically, the same year Rick was stricken with his mysterious illness, an extensive report issued by the Institute of Medicine (IOM), "Toxic Effects of Fungi and Bacteria" stated: "Occupants of damp and moldy buildings have sometimes reported central nervous system symptoms—such as fatigue, headache, memory loss, depression, and mood swings—that they attribute to the indoor environment. However, mycotoxin exposure of those people in their environment has not been identified and measured."[57] Nor had much research been conducted on humans, except for a small number of cancer studies.

Continuing research into mycotoxic illnesses demonstrates mold's ability to ignite an inflammatory response in genetically susceptible people. If you suspect mold may be at the root of your symptoms, authorities recommend a comprehensive mold inspection of your residence and worksite. Additionally, your automobile has its own ecosystem and can also be another potential source of mold contamination.

Food Storage and Cooking Options

Studies have found that certain chemicals in plastic that have been linked to health problems can leach into the food and drinks we consume. The leaching process can occur even faster when plastic is exposed to heat such as when microwaving leftovers in a plastic container.

Several chemicals in plastics, even at low doses, can be harmful when exposure occurs over the long term. Dr. Russ Hauser, chair of the Department of Environmental Health at the Harvard T.H. Chan School of Public Health, states:

> "We're talking about very low-dose chemical exposures. But even though single exposures to a specific chemical are small, if they occur repeatedly over long periods of time, their effects may add up, leading to a variety of adverse health outcomes down the road. Furthermore, and most importantly, we are exposed to many chemicals simultaneously (i.e. chemical mixtures) that may have additive adverse effects."[58]

Until more research confirms plastic's safety, it is best to choose glass or products other than plastic for both storage and cooking. Additionally, when using the microwave, use waxed paper instead of plastic wrap to cover food during cooking. I wish I had known 20 years earlier that plastic wrap also leaches toxins into food!

Ceramic cookware is a popular choice for nonstick cooking because it is safe under high heat, even when damaged. Ceramic cookware is fired in a kiln, making it durable and less prone to damage, then dipped in a glaze providing stain resistance and a nonstick coating. The ceramic coating applied on ceramic pots and pans does not contain dangerous PFOA or PTFE, once used in Teflon cookware. Teflon has been PFOA-free since 2013 and is now considered safe for normal home cooking.[59]

Electromagnetic Frequency Radiation (EMFs)

We the undersigned, more than 180 scientists and doctors from 35 countries, recommend a moratorium on the rollout of the fifth generation, 5G, for telecommunication until potential hazards for human health and the environment have been fully investigated by scientists independent from industry. 5G will substantially increase exposure to radiofrequency electromagnetic fields (RF-EMF) on top of the 2G, 3G, 4G, Wi-Fi, etc. for telecommunications already in place. RF-EMF has been proven to be harmful for humans and the environment.[60]

Signatories:
180 scientists from 35 nations
(99 scientists from European Union and 72 from other nations)

It was noted that a $25 million study by the National Toxicology Program (NTP), shows statistically significant increase in the incidence of brain and heart cancer in animals exposed to EMF below the ICNIRP (International Commission on Non-Ionizing Radiation Protection) guidelines followed by most countries. These results support results in human epidemiological studies on RF radiation and brain tumor risk. A large number of peer-reviewed scientific reports demonstrate harm to human health from EMFs.[61]

While wireless industries around the globe are racing to install 5G technologies, there has been a rigorous groundswell of science documenting significant health risks associated with exposure to radiofrequency radiation from cell phones, computers, and other modern wireless telecom devices.

Experts and government agencies continue to disagree about whether radiofrequency waves have a negative impact on our health and safety. Although many scientists have voiced their concerns regarding serious health risks from EMF exposure, those who love the convenience of connection but have not yet investigated the health risks, might not be so willing to embrace this next generation. While the future of 5G's global expansion is being explored, we are being exposed to existing EMFs from many devices.

The reality is that EMF-emitting devices have become convenient fixtures today, and convenience and connection are a priority for many. However, implementing some "EMF hygiene" helps to minimize exposure:[62]

- **Use a speakerphone or handset.** When using your cell phone, your safest bet is to talk through the speaker while holding the phone away from your head. The second choice is using is a wired headset.

- **Go "BlueTube," not BlueTooth**. As recommended by scientists concerned about EMFs, avoid using EMF-based Bluetooth-type headsets or earbuds, which increase exposure. Instead, use hard-wired headsets, or "BlueTube" headsets, utilizing plastic, stethoscope-like tubes to conduct soundwaves, but not EMF to the ear. Turn off your headset when not using your phone.

- **Use a case for your cellphone**. Since it is emitting radiation, carry your cell phone in a purse or briefcase rather than in a pocket or attached to a belt. Insert tablets and laptops in cases to reduce EMFs.

- **Use radiation blocking devices for your phone, computer, and other devices**.

- **Avoid placing a wireless device near your head while sleeping**. Place it at least six feet away.

- **Turn off your WIFI whenever it's not needed.** If using a wireless router, put it on a power strip for convenience and turn it off when not in use.

- **Limit your use of cell phones in enclosed spaces.** More radiation is emitted in cars, trains, planes, elevators, and enclosed metal spaces.

- **Opt to use wired appliances for your printer, computer, keyboard, and mouse.** Do this instead of wireless.

- **Avoid compact fluorescent (CFL) bulbs.** CFLs emit RF, UV and "dirty electricity" (a form of radio frequency (RF) radiation. It is everywhere, radiating through the walls in every room in your home, with irregular surges and spikes of electric energy moving along power lines and building wiring, where only standard 50 Hz to 60-Hz AC electricity should be. CFL bulbs contain mercury, and hazardous release of mercury if shattered. They must be disposed of as a toxic waste. Use energy efficient LED bulbs instead that do not generate RF or UV.

- **Say no to smart meters**. If a smart meter has been installed in your home, consider having it removed. Smart meters are not saving energy and they continually emit high intensity pulses—some meters pulse up to 190,000 times per day.

[W]e are creating a potential time bomb. If smart meters are placed in every home, they will contribute significantly to our exposure and this is both unwise and unsafe.[63]

Magda Havas, PhD,
professor of environmental and resource studies,
Trent University, Ontario, Canada

Personal Care, Cosmetics and Household Products

With heightened consumer awareness, industries are responding to the growing demand for products formulated with natural or organic ingredients. Consumers now have more choices but must continue reading labels to avoid hazardous ingredients.

Fortunately, the EWG has made shopping for cosmetics easier through its Skin Deep Guide® to Cosmetics. Additionally, it initiated the EWG Verified mark, assuring personal care, cosmetics and cleaning products meet its strict standards, and are free from EWG's chemicals of concern. As of 2020, more than 1,600 products have been approved for the EWG Verified mark.[64]

Water Filters

Water filtration systems remove many chemicals, pesticides, heavy metals, and bacterial contaminants, making water safer to drink, and often improving its taste. No filters or treatment systems are 100% effective in removing all contaminants from water so before you purchase one, you will need to know what contaminants you want to eliminate. Point-of-use water filters remove lead from drinking water immediately prior to consumption.

Different water filtration systems are available for either point-of-use or designed as a whole house system. Reverse osmosis filter systems are some of the strongest, most effective filters for drinking water. These have been tested to filter out 99% of the most dangerous contaminants, including heavy metals, herbicides, pesticides, chemicals, hormones, and other contaminants.

The quality of water in your area, listed by community and utility, is available through the Environmental Protection Agency. Each summer you should receive a Consumer Confidence Report (CCR), an annual drinking water quality report issued by your water supplier.[65] If your water is sourced from a well you can buy a home water quality kit, but the results may not be conclusive. You can find a list of labs recommended for every state or territory in the US at https://www.epa.gov/dwlabcert/contact-information-certification-programs-and-certified-laboratories-drinking-water.

Consult with Integrative Practitioners

Integrative, functional medicine: As highlighted in previous chapters, this medical model provides individualized, patient-centered, science-based approach to healthcare that empowers patients and practitioners to work together for addressing the underlying causes of disease and promotes optimal wellness. Functional medicine treatment targets the specific manifestations of disease in individuals. For more information and to find a practitioner, ifm.org/.

Integrative, biologically based dentistry: To a biological dentist, a healthy mouth is considered the gateway to whole body health, while a mouth teeming with toxicity, chronic infections, bacterial issues, poor root-canals, and other past procedures all have far reaching implications for full body health.

Biological dentists focus on preventing health problems including from toxic exposures in the mouth as well as materials often used in traditional dentistry. Recognizing the connection between a healthy oral microbiome and disease prevention, an integrative dentist offers specialized training for treating dental and mouth issues as well as providing preventative care for reducing the risks of chronic illness. More information about science-based biological dentistry is available at www.iaomt.org.

Making important changes requires a sustained and conscious commitment to your health. See the *Resources* section for pursuing additional resources for reducing toxicity and inflammation in support of vibrant health.

At no other time, have people, through reading and education, had such an important and crucial role in determining their own wellness.[66]

Sherry A. Rogers, MD

Chapter 21
A Wake Up Call for Us All

*Given the profound shifts in our gut microbiome created by an obsession
with being germ-free, the overuse of antibiotics, and the insidious
accumulation of toxins in our environment, we are all at risk of
becoming ill. What we are seeing is the tip of the proverbial iceberg.
Unless this problem is addressed—immediately—
we are all in trouble. All of us. No exceptions.*[1]

Neil Nathan, MD

With an estimated half of the population currently dealing with one or more chronic health conditions, we are seriously in need of a "wellness revolution." There are legions of people sick and tired of being sick and tired and who are desperately searching for the answers that conventional medicine has not been able to provide for transforming our collective health.

Patients often cope with similar consequences of chronic inflammatory illnesses—doctor visits that may take years to diagnose, exhaustive tests that do not pinpoint the root causes of inflammation, prescribed medications that do not heal while fueling adverse side effects, financial hardships, chronic stress, and—above all—the collapse of the way of life perhaps both patients and their loved ones once took for granted.

Globally, we are now well into 60 years of an intense toxic invasion, which has unleashed unprecedented, world-wide health issues. Distressing statistics project the skyrocketing trend of chronic illness and debilitation, spelling disaster for our bodies and brains.

Without building a new model, we are ultimately creating an ever-increasing patient load of disabled or debilitated citizens. Beyond the heartbreak of lives struck down from chronic illness, there is a collective economic hardship for us all. As the sickened are no longer able to work and may also require long-term care, fewer will be able to carry the burden. A nation sickened from policies, procedures, and products that are not protecting the safety of its citizens threatens colossal damage. Once you see the wisdom and superiority of a new reality, with the potential to transform our "sick care" model, you cannot return to an imperfect model.

Transforming Traditional Care

Today's conventional healthcare system cannot continue addressing 21st century health issues with the 20th century model of primarily treating symptoms without revealing their causes. Epidemiologic medicine deals with the incidence, distribution, and control of diseases. This approach does not recover wellness; it just suspends millions in a state of deteriorating health.

Chronic diseases account for 86% of healthcare costs, as noted on the Institute of Functional Medicine's website.[2] Conventional medicine is ideal for trauma cases and acute infections, but we need a seismic shift toward a holistic, integrative medical model that can also evaluate the root causes of chronic inflammation and resulting illnesses.

Conventional diagnostics and therapies that do not address root causes cannot help patients heal and recover. By embracing the diagnostics and therapies that have emerged from the field of integrative, functional medicine, practitioners can truly be emissaries of hope for patients stricken with neurodegenerative and other chronic inflammatory conditions.

Focus on Evolving Nutritional Science

> *The doctor of the future will no longer treat the human frame with drugs, but rather will cure and prevent disease with nutrition.*[3]
>
> Thomas Edison

The enlightened wisdom of Thomas Edison's reflections will prove transformational as science embraces a nutritional revolution. The microbiome is at the epicenter of revolutionary science and research, offering a new foundation for medicine. As we learn more about the intricacies of the microbiome, the future of healthcare can be predictive, personalized, preventative, and participatory—meaning people can directly impact their current and future health with proper nutrition and by adopting positive lifestyle choices.

Nutrigenomics, the study of the effects of food and food constituents on gene expression, continues to explore how genetic variations affect the nutritional environment.[4] Nutrigeneticists' continuing research will reveal greater awareness of the interaction between nutrients and genes and how this affects human health. Medical science must embrace new, innovative concepts to adequately study the effects of nutrition on health maintenance and disease prevention. It must translate the complex relationship between nutrition and health, respective to the genomic revolution.[5]

Down the road, if we could assess a person's gut microbial landscape and signaling molecules generated in this system, we could determine his or her vulnerability to antibiotics, stress, diet, and other destabilizing factors and design personalized treatments that could prevent the development of diseases, or restore the gut microbiome to health—through lifestyle modifications, dietary interventions, or future medical therapies.[6]

Emeran Mayer, MD

Expand Insurance Coverage for Functional Testing and Treatment

Currently, most consultations with integrative practitioners are not covered by insurance, nor are their recommended therapies or lab work—just conventional practices. This puts an unfair financial burden on patients who may not have the resources for accessing insightful evaluations and treatment, placing them outside the realm of receiving needed services.

Integrative practitioners currently have the right tools to properly evaluate and treat patients and offer guidance for disease prevention, including biomarker tests, hormone evaluation, mold and heavy metals testing, detoxification, and nutritional evaluation. Many of these tests and treatments are considered experimental, although they have proven repeatedly to be effective in diagnostics and treatment. Many are not covered by insurance, keeping them out-of-reach for many people. Ironically, these medical tests constitute a fraction of the costs required for ongoing monitoring and treatment of patients with chronic or life-threatening illnesses.

Traditional blood tests, MRIs, CT scans, and other diagnostic tests typically ordered by conventional practitioners are not—in many cases—the right tools for evaluating symptoms related to chronic inflammatory illnesses. To get to the root of the growing number of inflammatory and autoimmune illnesses currently plaguing 21st century life, the right diagnostics must be used.

Review Existing Industry Regulations through a Filter of Safety and Wellness

We've entered a new frontier of science, and not enough people or regulatory agencies are paying attention.[7]

Florence Williams, journalist and author

Thanks to regulations and manufacturers in North America, regulators (often with the aid of consumer advocacy groups) have reduced exposures to lead, asbestos, tobacco, radon, organochlorine pesticides, benzene, and others. Through corporate social responsibility, safer alternatives are being developed.

"Green" chemistry is creating green products in support of reducing toxic exposure and greater acceptance of corporate social responsibility.

Yet, there is much more that needs to be done. We need to escalate the protection and safety of our food, water, air, and consumer products to both reduce and prevent the scourge of chronic illness and help reduce our national and international toxic burdens. We can advocate for this by what we choose to buy, and from which companies.

Approval processes of regulators must prevent the use of chemicals not proven safe or confirmed to be health hazards. Heavy metals are poisoning our air and water, being formulated into vaccines, and used as ingredients in everything from light bulbs to lipstick in consumer products while poisoning our bodies.

It is the continuing responsibility of regulators, committed to creating a national paradigm of wellness, to review national policies and regulations with health as the top priority and safeguard its citizens. By holding to the highest standards, consumer health and well-being must become the priority.

By restructuring all systems currently causing harm within interconnected regulatory agencies and industries, and the policies that shape them, we can begin to envision new horizons for healthier realities. Such a paradigm offers more than hope and requires action for all who contribute to the production and delivery of goods and services and the regulations that monitor them. The detoxing of our economy is not a focus of this book but is necessary to support the overall health for our nation.

Only when people exercise their power as both citizens and consumers
will there be solutions to the problems caused
by damaging chemicals in the environment.[8]
Bruce Lourie and Rick Smith, authors of *Toxin Toxout*

Better Health Destinies on the Horizon?

Healthy citizens are the greatest asset any country can have. [9]
Winston Churchill

Wellness is energizing! Its power ignites us into action to achieve our goals and pursue our passions. A nation filled with a strong, energized populace instinctively fires up a collective winning spirit of unlimited possibilities and innovations. In contrast, sickness is debilitating as it depletes our collective energy, initiative, and endurance. When a nation's citizenry is perpetually plagued with sickness and sapped of its life force, it is unable to fully deploy its most valuable asset—its people. We the people say "yes" to health!

The skyrocketing statistics across the spectrum of chronic diseases signal a critical need for adopting wellness wisdom with a relentless commitment. All parts of the health equation play decisive roles in our interconnected network for transforming our health destinies.

While personal responsibility largely shapes our own fate, so does our influence in modeling healthy habits to impact our family's wellness. Additionally, through both our voting and activism, we can help to shape policies aimed for maximizing health in our communities, in our businesses, and beyond. We have had many opportunities to witness how integrity and common sense have been compromised in decisions impacting health. By uniting with a collective health consciousness, the potential for leveraging desired changes exists.

Making vibrant wellness a national priority requires new initiatives within a consortium across all arenas, impacting health outcomes. Imagine what would manifest nationally through participation in a "Top Priority Health Commitment," a collective vision, mission, and purpose. This may sound unrealistic, yet if we are to create a nation of energized, healthy citizens, then participation of all parts related to the whole is essential.

Consider the positive impact from such a comprehensive initiative. The weaving together of medical schools, healthcare facilities, daycare, schools, policy makers, regulators, insurance companies, food producers, consumer product manufacturers, advertisers, media, and others is vital. It would help create an interconnected web of health promotion, production, environmental oversight, and more. It would promote and provide the healthiest of foods available at home, in restaurants, hospitals, and other institutions; offer environmentally safe products and systems to protect the environment; provide revolutionary healing modalities; promote inspiring messaging regarding positive lifestyle choices; and more. Adopting such a shared vision through uniting together would be transformational!

"Tick tock" goes the toxic clock. Much is now known regarding these critical interrelationships in support of health. It will be a daunting task to restructure personal habits, infrastructure systems, and policies which have contributed to the development and escalation of these horrific diseases.

Fortunately, there is movement in many directions, but for those currently suffering, it is not fast enough. Science is evolving, which is ushering new pathways for a paradigm of wellness, but we are not there ... yet. We still have a long way to go for incorporating essential changes into our current, flawed system of healthcare based on outdated science. However, the outlook appears promising.

In reference to biotoxin illnesses, what is now scientifically validated dwarfs the knowledge base when only Dr. Shoemaker's revolutionary science precisely pinpointed Rick's issues. As Dr. Shoemaker writes in *Surviving Mold: Life in the Era of Dangerous Buildings*: "Back in 2004, there was only the hope that opinions about mold illness written by U.S. government agencies and the World Health Organization would actually mirror what we knew then to be true... We now have clear evidence that shows that mold illness comes from exposure to the diverse mixture of compounds found in water damaged buildings (WDBs) and that the illness is based on the inflammation those compounds cause. Furthermore, it's inhaling those inflammagens (antigens, or foreign particles, that activate innate immune responses) that makes people sick, based on their genetic make-up."[10]

> *It is time to improve medical education in the field of*
> *chronic inflammatory responses syndromes for those*
> *who arrogantly deny the existence of mold illness.*[11]
>
> Ritchie Shoemaker, MD

Even with evolving science and recent breakthroughs in research, there are legions of patients right now, anxiously awaiting answers. When it comes to solutions, we cannot afford to linger. These illnesses are having a seismic impact on our society—physically, emotionally, mentally, spiritually, socially, and financially. Massive changes are required for addressing multiple issues associated with all the burdens of chronic inflammatory illnesses, not only for today's patients, but for millions more looming on the horizon. If changes are not made, they too will be seeking services in an ill-prepared healthcare system.

Surveying the current state of national health, alarming statistics should spur us into united action. None of us can accept the consequences of the status quo. We are all at risk, and those who are genetically wired are the first to fall. Multiple measures must be taken to avoid such madness, both in and beyond healthcare, and for all who will most assuredly suffer from these debilitating futures, if we do not make different choices.

Far too many people are still not yet aware of how much we individually determine our health destinies. Providing accurate health education to doctors and to the public is essential to realize how we can reduce our own risks of suffering an unwelcome fate. Ultimately, to experience vibrant wellness, we must wake up to the scientific realities contributing to neurodegenerative and other inflammatory illnesses. Once underlying causes are addressed, the mystery causing them is unveiled. Destinies will be changed.

Time is ticking. Time to reduce toxic impact upon our citizens. Time for more training. Time for better testing and therapies. Waste no more time to educate and train doctors, arming them with the right tools and technologies for 21st century illnesses.

Individually, as well as collectively, we can shift the paradigm so greater wellness for all is our destiny. Time for us all to recognize our power to support our own wellness and embrace healthcare options that deliver dynamic destinies!

In the meantime, since there are now many options available for evaluation and treatment, we must do our own due diligence in exploring our health concerns. Seek health professionals who offer a focus on prevention and recovery of your issues rather than just treating or masking symptoms. Time is a critical factor in both prevention and healing.

We must come together to do this. We must reach out, talk with one another and reestablish real connections to begin this process of neurological rebooting on a planetary level ... I pray that all of you will help in this healing effort. Our lives, and the lives of our children and grandchildren, depend on it.[12]

Neil Nathan, MD

Chapter 22
An Evolving Renaissance in Brain Wellness

Currently, with soaring statistics painting a dismal future for those stricken with debilitating brain disorders and other diseases, a revitalization of the healthcare industry is desperately needed. Fortunately, science continues to reveal more solutions, and the landscape of brain health is transforming with new understandings and emerging innovations.

Dedicated doctors sharing their insights with other doctors is accelerating both the treatment and prevention of cognitive decline for patients, such as Dr. Bredesen's revolutionary protocol programs: PreCODE (to optimize brain health and prevent cognitive decline) and ReCODE (reversing cognitive decline). These programs include a thorough evaluation with recommendations for correcting imbalances to optimize patient health and a proven pathway for preventing or reversing cognitive decline.

These programs are personalized to the patient's needs, based on the laboratory values found to be abnormal. They address the root cause or the prevention of an abnormality rather than just focusing upon a single therapy. Both are comprehensive, customized plans related to needed dietary changes, detoxification, supplements, healing the gut, exercise, stress reduction, brain training, enhancing sleep, balancing hormones, among other adjustments to optimize a patient's wellness.[1] (Dr. Watts is receiving certification in the ReCODE protocol.)

Bredesen's protocols have generated extensive proof of their effectiveness. In the study published in 2021, "Precision Medicine Approach to Alzheimer's Disease: Successful Proof-of-Concept Trial" included 25 participants, aged 50 to 76, all with MCI (pre-Alzheimer's) or early-stage dementia. Each patient was assessed for multiple potential contributors — inflammation, insulin resistance, nutrient and hormonal deficiencies, specific pathogens, toxicants, and biotoxins, as well as genetics — then treated with a personalized protocol that was continued for nine months. Cognitive testing revealed that among the study participants, 21 improved (84%), one showed no change (4%), and three declined (12%).[2] An 84% improvement!

These positive results support the premise that identifying and treating the contributors to cognitive decline with a personalized protocol for each patient, represents an effective treatment approach for patients with mild cognitive impairment or early dementia. They offer new horizons for conquering dementia with science-based solutions. These protocols provide exciting prospects for those experiencing dementia or mild cognitive impairment, as well as those at risk due to family histories of dementia.

While Dr. Bredesen's protocols are focused on the three different types of Alzheimer's including type 3 (toxic), Rick's illness exhibited a combination of that type and Lewy body dementia. As Dr. Bredesen notes, " ... we do have examples of Lewy body disease with documented improvement, and the evaluations of patients with Lewy body disease suggest that it is related to type 3 (toxic) Alzheimer's disease, in that high levels of toxins (metallotoxins, organic toxins, or biotoxins) are typically present."[3]

In Dr. Bredesen's 2021 book, *The First Survivors of Alzheimer's,* initial participants in his revolutionary program, share their transformational stories, detailing the fear, struggle, and ultimate victory of each of their journeys, offering hope for everyone with the potential for dramatic changes in health destinies.

These two entries by Kristin, the first patient in the Bredesen Protocol program reflects the power of these transformational interventions:

> *I know that I am on that slippery slope into Alzheimer's and I am terrified. My short-term memory is gone. Thoughts fly out of my head seconds after they form. I cant deny or hide it any longer. I feel lost ...*
> Kristin's Journal entry, 2011

***

10 years later ... 2021

> *Dr. Bredesen developed the road map. I follow it ... I owe my life to Dr. Bredesen, and I will be eternally grateful to him and for the incredible work he has done to bring an end to Alzheimer's for so many people. Bredesen's work sheds light in the dungeon of despair where people with Alzheimer's reside.[4]*
> Kristin, age 77
> *The First Survivors of Alzheimer's*

In addition to the continuing expansion of functional medicine for precision evaluation and treatment, a plethora of research validates the promise of energy medicine. This is defined as "any energetic or informational interaction with a biological system to bring back homeostasis in the organism."

Scientists are rapidly discovering that the human body is indeed a complex electromagnetic field, immersed in other intricate environmental, electromagnetic frequencies and light waves. These all serve as a "control center" for our physical and mental performance. When those energy fields become blocked or disrupted, that sets the stage for health issues to arise. Removing those blocks in the body's energetic field is the basis of energy medicine. [5]

The future of medicine is understanding the crucial relationship between the material and "field" aspects of the body, and adjusting human frequencies—and light, sound and electromagnetic interventions are crucial here—to prevent illness and boost health.[6]

Joanne De Luca and Janine Lopiano,
co-founders of Sputnik Futures, a future-forecasting consultancy

Physicists recognize our entire world is electrodynamic, with effects rising from the interactions of rapidly changing electric and magnetic fields. Both natural and man-made frequencies impact human cells. As Beth McGroarty reported in "Energy Medicine Gets Serious," summarizing the forecast of energy medicine at the 2020 Global Wellness Summit: "We're at a most remarkable moment in time, where the medical world and 'ancient wellness' are finding some common (at least in principle) theoretical ground. Science is continuing to validate some crucial ancient energy medicine principles."[7]

Once viewed with skepticism for those unaware of the power of energy medicine, it has been validated in more than 600 research studies, including such therapies as acupuncture, reiki, craniosacral therapy, and many others. The National Institute for Integrative Healthcare (NIIH) is a leading-edge nonprofit dedicated to research and education in the fields of energy medicine and energy psychology. It investigates the epigenetic effects of intention, consciousness, and energy in healing (describing the influences that alter the expression of genes from outside the gene). Research projects have demonstrated that consciousness (beliefs, emotions, optimism, altruism, visualization, prayer, energy, and meditation) have epigenetic effects, affecting cellular processes at the most fundamental levels of molecular biology.[8]

The rapidly expanding field of energy medicine offers a wide variety of technologies, offering more than hope for healing with positive, proven outcomes. With a multitude of studies relative to healing the brain, in the following section I've cited just a few of these modalities as an illustration for the potential healing for brain health.

Low level light therapy (LLLT): Let there be light! This is an essential element of life, as we are light-dependent beings. Evolving science has engineered beneficial red and near-infrared wavelengths, colors of the sun's light, into LLLT technology, also known as photobiomodulation (PBM). This term was established in 2016 as a medical science heading, used by the National Institutes of Health as part of its published research database to describe this emerging science. Light technology continues to gain recognition from authorities in medical schools, scholarly journals, medical practitioners, therapists, and others concerned with biomedical science.[9]

Largely propelled by progress in the fields of photobiology and bioenergetics, these light frequencies have demonstrated compelling beneficial physiological effects. Research demonstrates that PBM signals damaged cells to begin their repair processes. The light energy is soaked up by the mitochondria, the "power generators" of cells, helping to repair and create healthier ones. This is a photo-chemical response, not a heat/thermal response, so the tissue is safe from thermal damage.

Light therapy has proven efficacious with many different diseases, conditions, and fields of medical treatment including neurological, memory, mood and ophthalmic disorders, wound healing, fatigue, arthritis, and an expanding list of others.[10]

In a small research study, brain-injured patients received near-infrared light therapy with participants reporting better memory, sleep, and mood. Additionally, neuropsychological testing before and through monitoring and follow-up, showed gains in executive function, verbal learning, and memory.[11]

In another study, veterans were assessed for the impact of light therapy upon their Gulf War Illness symptoms, traumatic brain injury, and PTSD. Researchers applied red and near-infrared light, using a specially designed helmet. Light therapy boosts the output of nitric oxide near the location of the LEDs, improving blood flow in that area, as was shown on MRI scans. It had measurable effect on damaged brain cells, specifically on their mitochondria. The red and near-infrared light photons penetrate through the skull and into brain cells, stimulating the mitochondria to produce more ATP. "That can mean clearer, sharper thinking," said lead investigator Dr. Margaret Naeser. She envisions light therapy potential for other brain-related conditions including depression, stroke, dementia, and autism.[12]

Optogenetics: This is a branch of biotechnology that combines genetics and optical techniques to conceive and control specific neural circuits in the brain. This offers neurobiologists a vital mapping of the brain's connections to activate or silence certain brain circuits. Optogenetics can be applied to study numerous disorders that arise in the brain and is anticipated to be able to treat many neurological conditions.[13]

Craniosacral therapy: A gentle, hands-on method of evaluating and enhancing the functioning of the craniosacral system, comprised of the membranes and cerebrospinal fluid that surround and protect the brain and spinal cord. Cumulative research continues to demonstrate its effectiveness in treating Alzheimer's and dementias, closed head injuries, autism, cerebral palsy, concussion, headaches, and more.

The CranioSacral System was first described by Dr. John Upledger, an osteopath and researcher who developed the corresponding therapy in the 1970s. Upledger's research revealed that, as we age, the circulation of cerebrospinal fluid decreases by as much as 50%, from the aging process, inflammation of the brain, head trauma or injury, accumulation of heavy metals, or other conditions.

> *Exercising the cranial therapy system enhances the ability to flush unwanted toxic materials from the brain and spinal cord tissues. Since it is now known that cerebrospinal fluid carries small, metal-chelating molecules, clearly the enhanced flushing may remove unwanted metallic deposits from the brain and spinal fluid tissues.*[14]
>
> John Upledger, DO, OMM

In 2012, a team of neuroscientists identified the glymphatic system, named for the glial cells that play a key role in managing the waste removal and regulation of the brain tissues. The glymphatic system pushes large volumes of cerebrospinal fluid through the brain along specific pathways. As it flows through the brain, the cerebrospinal fluid collects proteins and other debris and carries it to lymphatic ducts, thereby clearing the brain of waste. Some of these waste products are amyloid ß, a type of protein that is continuously produced and secreted from brain cells and linked to Alzheimer's disease. When these critical pathways fail from aging, injury, inflammation, or infection in the brain, the restricted flow of cerebrospinal fluid cause the withering of those regions deprived of the life-giving fluid.[15]

Additional research at the Upledger Institute, headed by Michael Morgan LMT, CST-D, discovered that in those people diagnosed with senile dementia, the flow of cerebrospinal fluid was decreased by 75% in comparison to a healthy adult. Morgan notes that the decrease in the volume of cerebrospinal fluid leads to brains drying up during the aging process, resulting in an accumulation of toxins and restrictions in the brain, including the amyloid plaques and neurofibrillary tangles associated with Alzheimer's disease.[16]

With knowledge of the vital importance of the glymphatic system in removing waste from the body and the brain, craniosacral therapy offers proven pathways for wellness in treating dementias and other disorders.

Sound therapy: With the emergence of encephalography and its ability to record the electrical activity of the brain, researchers have studied brainwave patterns and how they respond to external stimuli. A vast body of data shows therapeutic application of sound to modulate brainwave patterns, affect sympathetic-parasympathetic balance, and synchronize the activity of the left and right brain hemispheres.

Dr. Jeffrey Thompson, director of the Center for Neuroacoustic Research in San Diego, has been exploring how our brains interpret sounds and the therapeutic application of sound for more than 20 years. His work is based on two key principles: 1) that every tissue, just like every physical object, will resonate to very specific sound frequencies; and 2) that there are mechanisms within the nervous system that synchronize neurophysiologic functions and cycles with coherent, rhythmic pulsations from the external world: "It is akin to the picking of a lock on the neurophysiologic processes that the body already uses to heal itself."[17]

Dr. Thompson also reports: "Using sound in these ways, it is possible to make profound changes in brainwave patterns and states of consciousness, observable on brainwave mapping equipment (EEG), as well as positive changes in the body, measurable with blood tests, biofeedback equipment and other sophisticated procedures. We are also able to influence the core balance and functioning of the brain and central nervous system as a whole."[18]

Sound healing through music and its effects on brain chemistry has been widely researched, with a review of some 400 published scientific articles. The rhythmic stimulation of music has proven to have a significant impact in reducing pain as well as providing many other mental and physical health benefits in managing mood and stress.[19]

Genetic Therapies: Research into the realms of genetic engineering offer exciting prospects of powerful epigenetic future therapies. This will be welcome news for patients afflicted with brain diseases and all conditions whenever this capability is ultimately incorporated into standard care.

With regards to brain issues, this is especially relevant for those with poor detoxifying genes, as described earlier as a key factor of Rick's illness. When the methylation process is genetically compromised, it has been linked to autoimmune, neurological, and other inflammatory conditions. Research has targeted DNA methylation, which shows promise in improving this critical process in future therapeutic applications.[20]

Scientists have already figured out how to modify the epigenome, allowing researchers to turn off almost any gene in human cells to prevent its expression, without making a single edit to the genetic code. Once a gene is switched off, it remains inert in the cell's descendants for hundreds of generations.

Jennifer Doudna, PhD, a professor of chemistry, biochemistry, and molecular biology at UC Berkeley forecast in late 2020: "Within 30 years, it will probably be possible to make essentially any kind of change to any kind of genome," … in the future, we're not subject to the DNA we inherit from our parents but we can actually change our genes in a targeted way."[21] This means your DNA doesn't define your destiny!

Indeed, the winds of change are carrying new healing technologies our way. We are at a pivotal, powerful moment in time, with a world of possibilities from advancements in science and energy medicine. Oh, what wonderful things await us on the horizon! Imagine a world of wellbeing that could be offered with frequencies for quantum healing therapy—precision diagnostics, surgical repairs, DNA support, and rejuvenation without the need for toxic chemicals, medications, or processes linked to side effects. Both science and new technologies are expanding the realms of healing possibilities, heralding new dimensions in wellness.

I embrace a collective vision of wellness and wellbeing shifting dramatically across the global landscape—availability of safe, precise, affordable, accessible diagnostics, treatment, and prevention care for all. We eagerly anticipate the time when this paradigm shift manifests these new realities for preventing and treating not only neurological issues, but for all conditions that diminish our health. Our future is now ripe with once unimagined possibilities emerging and evolving, leading us to gratefully experience a destiny of vibrant wellness!

> *In the coming years, there will be a rush by medical and technology companies to further crack the code on how energy networks organize our bodies and brains, and they will use that knowledge to design interventions into our electromagnetic and biophotonic fields to prevent disease and boost physical and mental health. It will create entirely new medical approaches, new products and new business models.*[22]
> Beth McGroarty, *2020 Global Wellness Trends*

Part 5

Strategies for Managing Life's Uncertainties

Chapter 23
Managing the Collateral Chaos from Chronic Illness

Our journey would not be complete without sharing my perspectives as a caregiver, a role I never anticipated would transform my life in every possible way. Loved ones are typically thrust into these roles and are quite unprepared for all the challenges they will face when a family member develops a chronic, debilitating illness. Especially for those managing loved ones with brain issues, on-the-job training is inadequate for an extended duration of round-the-clock care. This section describes the collateral damage related to long-term illness, and the strategies that helped to sustain me through the most challenging period of my life.

We are never fully prepared for the many challenges created by a chronic illness or disability. The chronically ill, robbed of their physical health and vitality, often suffer losses in other areas of their lives, including their careers, finances, relationships, and overall quality of life, adding to the stress level and tensions throughout the family unit.

Due to the loss of income from the stricken partner or spouse's disability, adjustments are required for the other to serve not only as caregiver, but often in the dual capacity as breadwinner. When prolonged illnesses endure, the combination of loss of income, mounting medical bills, and expensive care costs can drain life savings and drive many into bankruptcy. Combined into this costly mixture are concerns and tensions related to their care, safety, and welfare, along with the well-being for all members of the family. Caregiver's stress mounts for anyone handling it all, who often question their ability to sustain their own spirits and strength through a siege of unknown duration.

Preplanning can avert some of the practical issues that arise with debilitating illness, but it is also critical to develop other inner-focused strategies that emphasize self-care and the power of positive attitudes for navigating the inevitable challenges inherent with chronic illnesses.

Preparing for the Unexpected

Before Rick's illness struck, we were focused on our careers, college plans for our daughters, future travel plans, and the typical day-to-day concerns of a busy modern family. We were both self-employed; fortunately, Rick had secured both short and long-term disability policies for himself. To me, a "disability" was a remote possibility—I could not envision anything striking us that could be that disabling and life-changing. Indeed, my optimistic spirit was especially grateful for Rick's more practical nature.

A conversation with one of my friends who had been stricken with cancer awakened me to the unexpected turns that life can suddenly take. She urged us to secure long-term care insurance and Rick and I scheduled a meeting with her agent immediately. We purchased long-term care coverage, choosing the option to share care from each other's policy, in case either one of us exhausted his or her own.

We also had other important legal documents prepared for one another: the previously mentioned power of attorney (POA), healthcare POA, and our wills. You cannot plan for every contingency, but having these legal documents, along with insurance policies for short and long-term disability, and long-term care insurance, proved to be life savers for us when the unimaginable happened.

Creating Your ICE File

Having an "In Case of Emergency" (ICE) file is an essential organizational tool when disaster strikes for any reason. We did not prepare ours in advance, but I wasted no time once Rick's illness became apparent.

Under most circumstances, having the POA and the healthcare POA documents in place will be sufficient for handling the financial, legal, and health management concerns if a loved one is stricken. Preplanning can also avoid the conflicts that may arise when family members disagree on health management and the financial and legal responsibilities for care.

In addition, your ICE file should include other critical documents, e.g., Social Security numbers; employment, military, and tax records; bank and investment accounts; and any other financial or personal documents, maintained in a secure place.

If your responsibilities will include parents or other loved ones, you will need to compile similar documents for them as described below. While it may be uncomfortable talking about matters of money, mortality, wills, and wishes, it is a necessary conversation.

Power of Attorney: A POA allows you to designate someone you trust to make financial, tax, and legal decisions on your behalf should you become incapacitated. With a POA, your designated legal representative can manage your financial affairs, sell property, pay bills, make deposits, discuss your insurance policies, and serve as payee for your Social Security payments, among other decisions.

Ordinary POA vs. Durable POA: There is a critical difference between an ordinary POA and a durable POA. An ordinary POA can be revoked by you at any time while you have the legal capacity to act. If you become injured, sick, disabled, or unable to communicate, an ordinary POA is no longer legally effective. A durable POA can be drafted so that the POA becomes effective immediately and continues for the duration of your sickness or disability or can specify that it becomes effective only when you become incapacitated. A durable POA maintains your representative's legal rights to serve on your behalf.

As the principal, you can legally revoke a durable POA at any time unless you become incapacitated. When this happens, as it did after my husband revoked my ability to serve in that capacity, I had to provide evidence of his incapacitation to the court so I could be appointed his guardian and conservator. Only after guardianship and conservatorship were granted was I legally permitted to again manage all his financial, legal, and care concerns.

Advanced Health Care Directive: This includes two documents: 1) a healthcare POA, which designates a person you authorize to make medical decisions on your behalf in the event you become incapacitated. A HIPAA release gives your representative the authority to access your health records and doctors; and 2) a "living will" outlining the type of care you want to receive if you become incapacitated. This could include a Do Not Resuscitate Order (DNR) or a preference for comfort care only.

Additional Documents: Assemble all your important documents and notify a trusted friend or relative of their location. Ideally, you should keep originals in a safe deposit box or fireproof box with copies safely stored at home. Review these with your spouse, partner, adult children, or other responsible party and update, as necessary. Documents should include:

- Insurance policies
- Wills and living trusts
- Bank accounts
- Investment accounts
- Credit card information
- Birth and marriage certificates
- Social Security numbers
- Employment, military, and tax records
- Real estate deeds and car titles

- Passwords
- Burial preferences and funeral arrangements
- Contact numbers of your attorney, doctors, financial advisor, insurance agent, the location of your safe deposit box and keys, and other information that might be necessary.

The Priceless Value of Insurance

Long-Term Disability Insurance

Disability insurance provides a portion of your income if you become too sick or hurt to return to work. Although Rick wanted desperately to continue working after the onset of his illness, his diminished cognitive abilities prevented him from doing so. Fortunately, he had purchased long-term disability insurance years before his illness struck. Without this policy, our family's financial situation would have been disastrous.

Long-Term Care Insurance

Our long-term care insurance policies turned out to be the best investment we ever made. With Rick's sometimes frightening behavioral issues he could no longer be cared for at home. The cost of his care would have been financially devastating and emotionally draining for our family.

Timing for securing long-term care insurance is critical. Pre-existing conditions can either make the cost prohibitive or disqualify you altogether. Ideally, you should buy the policies while you and your loved one are still healthy. If you need further incentive to justify what will seem like a costly investment, I suggest you research the cost per month of a skilled nursing care unit. In 2020, the median monthly cost for a semi-private room was nearly $7,800 and rising annually.[1]

Another smart choice we made in exploring plans was selecting the shared care option. This allows a married couple to take out separate plans, which offer an option allowing each spouse to become a "rider" on their partner's plan. The shared benefit rider gives a couple a pool of benefits to split between them. During his twelve-year illness, Rick exhausted his own long-term coverage after ten years. Fortunately, I had purchased another policy in 2005 for myself, just in case. That proved to be another wise strategic move with his long-term illness.

Chapter 24
Caregiving and Care Issues

Caring for a person with dementia also means managing symptoms that caregivers of people with other diseases may not face, such as neuropsychiatric symptoms (for example, anxiety, apathy, and lack of inhibition) and severe behavioral problems.[1]
Alzheimer's Association

For those stricken with a neurological condition, caregiving options are a big concern. When ailing adults can no longer manage their own affairs, responsibility usually shifts to family members, who are typically not prepared for all its demands. Only 9% of those between the ages of 55 and 70 have planned to pay for a caregiver when they need such help. This puts a tremendous strain on caregivers.

In 2020, approximately 15.3 million family members and friends provided unpaid care to people with Alzheimer's and other dementias, at an economic value of $256.7 billion. Fifty-seven percent of family caregivers of people with Alzheimer's and related dementias provide care for four years or more.[2]

The responsibility of caregiving, which often falls to a partner or children, is a daunting task, one filled with inconceivable challenges. The Alzheimer's Association reports that four out of five caregivers want more help from family, and battles among adult siblings are among the most common sources of friction regarding care responsibilities for a parent stricken with dementia. Families that divide responsibilities typically manage better without festering resentments, e.g., taking responsibility for managing finances and paying bills, driving the person to medical appointments, grocery shopping, hands-on care, and others. Online resources are available to help families in all 50 states locate government, nonprofit, and private caregiver support programs.[3]

According to the Alzheimer's Association, the average lifetime cost of care for a person with Alzheimer's was nearly $375,000 in 2020, a financial burden that is mounting annually. Seventy percent of the lifetime cost of care is borne by family caregivers, which includes the value of unpaid caregiving, as well as out-of-pocket expenses for medications, food, and others costs for individuals with dementia. Financial burdens for necessary care are a grim reality, not to mention the incalculable toll upon the emotional, physical, and mental wellbeing of caregivers.[4]

Over the course of Rick's illness, options for respite and long-term care offered invaluable support including some of these:

Respite Care

Respite care is a service that provides either temporary or long-term care for a loved one requiring assistance. It supports family caregivers by relieving them of their duties so they can rest and recharge. **In-home or companion care** is offered by someone from outside the home who assists with activities of daily living (ADLs), such as bathing, dressing, eating, or minor household chores, such as laundry and meals.

- **Live-in caregivers** can be either temporary or permanent. Professional aides or home health aides are available through government or community agencies. Temporary caregivers allow family members to take a break from caregiving responsibilities for a short time, while permanent live-in caregivers provide long-term ongoing care. No matter who will be serving as the caregiver, make sure that they are aware of behaviors associated with the loved one's illness, particularly those with specific forms of dementia.

- **Adult day care** offers daytime supervision for patients with dementia and disabilities. Meals, snacks, supervision, activities, and personal care assistance is provided. It is a great care option for caregivers who work part or full-time; some centers offer transportation to and from the adult daycare facility.

- **Residential respite care** (short-term overnight) provides professional, residential care up to several weeks in hospitals, nursing homes, assisted living facilities, and group homes.

Long-Term Care

Every day until 2030, some 10,000 Baby Boomers will turn 65—seven out of ten people will require long-term care in their lifetimes.[5]

- **Assisted Living** offers disabled or infirm adults a continuum of services related to housing, personal care, healthcare and enrichment activities for those who cannot or choose not to live independently. Services include assistance as required for ADLs, e.g., eating, dressing, grooming, mobility, and toileting.

- **Skilled Nursing Care** provides residential care for people needing help with daily activities and supervised with professional medical care.

When It's Time to Take Away Car Keys

With keys to the car, I soon realized the dangers associated with Rick's mental impairment were jeopardizing his safety as well as others on the road. Rick never would have considered risking the safety of others before his illness robbed him of his good sense.

If a loved one shows signs of impairment behind the wheel, it is time to act for the safety of all concerned. If the impaired driver does not recognize these deficiencies, he or she is unlikely to willingly hand over the keys.

Losing the ability to drive is a major loss of self-sufficiency and freedom, and the reason giving up a driver's license can create ferocious conflicts, as it did for us. According to the Alzheimer's Association, families often delay taking away the keys, knowing it is a battle zone, but that has the potential for dangerous consequences.

The best way to assess if it's time to take away the keys is to have the suspected impaired driver tested by an occupational therapist or an organization with specific training and experience in evaluating driver safety. If the person fails the evaluation, third-party testing provides needed evidence regarding safety. This also eliminates the family member being wedged into an uncomfortable role in a potentially hostile situation. Speaking from experience, I cannot emphasize this enough!

Developing a Resilient Spirit

Prior to my husband's illness, I had written books and training manuals and presented seminars about the power of resiliency and winning attitudes in transforming even the most tragic life situations. For decades I had researched case histories and interviewed countless indomitable spirits who overcame their seemingly insurmountable circumstances. Their unshakable desire to create a different reality did exactly that, illustrating the power of inspiring attitudes.

In retrospect, this served as my own personal development course as I would soon have to draw on that wisdom for all the challenges that lay ahead. The 12-year experience of navigating my husband's neurological issues tested my fortitude to remain steadfast while meeting life's challenges with courage, strength, and wisdom. I had to come to terms with letting go of the life I had anticipated and finding joy in the life I was living.

That idea is not just a platitude, but hard-won wisdom from my time in the trenches during Rick's illness. When I looked around and saw my friends moving toward their goals, by contrast our future seemed littered with dead ends. I was feeling overburdened and anxious as endless responsibilities gobbled up my time, energy, and resources. Ironically, as a motivational speaker who encouraged people to adopt an attitude of gratitude, I became painfully aware of not always being able to "walk my talk."

Giving voice to my worry periodically, and briefly, was both cathartic and therapeutic. I tried not to dwell on the multiple fears that would arise in facing new issues—a key component for finding balance and sanity throughout the turbulence of my new reality. When I noticed unwelcome, unproductive feelings rising, I did my best to shift them to align with my goal, which was a peaceful, happy heart.

I am a big proponent of the "Law of Attraction"—simply stated, whatever you give the most attention, be it positive or negative, is what you will continue to attract into your life. It's a compelling reason to let go of thoughts that don't reflect what you most desire. I had to monitor both my inner and outer conversations to avoid "awfulizing" situations that only made the situation worse, such as, "This is so devastating for us!" or, "How awful that this illness has made such a mess of our lives." I did not deny my feelings of being overwhelmed. I just acknowledged them and replaced them with thoughts that uplifted my spirit.

As someone who embraces intentional living, I focused on what I desired and intended to experience by using daily affirmations to manifest my vison. "Nothing can disturb the calm peace of my soul," was one I uttered countless times a day to shift me back to a more peaceful heart. Another verse from the wisdom of the poem, *Desiderata*, served as a reminder to release and let go: "And whether or not it is clear to you, no doubt the universe is unfolding as it should. Therefore, be at peace."[6]

Never navigate such a journey alone! A wise friend counseled me early on to accept help from those who offered it. As an independent woman who prided herself on handling it all, I learned the value of being specific as to what I needed and asking for it. Fortunately, I had a circle of caring souls who bolstered my spirits throughout Rick's illness, providing me a space for expressing my angst and fears. They reminded me that at my core, I was strong, capable, wise, and resilient.

A light-hearted spirit focused upon intentional living and resilience can get you through the toughest of times. By adapting to the changes required, your resilience will empower you in re-engineering your life around new circumstances. How you show up in this new role can be both a blessing and an inspiration to others and make navigating the course easier.

Accept what is, let go of what was, and let your resilient spirit soar!

Part 6

Navigating with Heart

Reflections

While I have shared my reflections throughout the years of Rick's illness, it seemed fitting to include a few of Rick's own sentiments, in his own words. Sometimes his brain worked well; at other times, he escaped into a world I could not access. Much of the time, it was hard to know what Rick was thinking, and there were periods as well in which he was unable to communicate much at all.

It was a journey of body, mind, and heart, with transformations of all three through this agonizing process. For a long time, his journal entries centered around the tenuous nature of his physical condition and what was causing such confusion and agony. Suspended in a state of not knowing, he often questioned his destiny.

By nature, Rick was an observant soul and monitoring many present moments, offering us a glimpse into that painful reality for an extended endurance run of faith.

In his own words

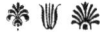

By writing out my thoughts offers a brief displacement of mental energy and a focus beyond the physical. If anyone ever wants to know what I'm experiencing, they can read my ramblings. Maybe there's a purpose in doing so.

"Wherever I am, God is, and all is well." That's a tough one right now in the condition I'm in. I ask for peace of spirit and for serenity within my body, believing healing is possible. I listen for answers and await healing.

What am I supposed to do now? I linger in a body that no longer works well. It takes all my energy sometimes to move, and then I question, for what? I have been waiting an inordinate amount of time for any answers. Special people have come into my life, but not one as of now have had solutions.

What is this existence of myself now? What is the lesson? I ask and ask and pray but continue to suffer.

Where is the spiritual hearing aid? Where is the compassion to allow such suffering? Yes, I am aware of others suffering, perhaps from the same unexplainable causes of an illness not recognized, at least not yet. Did I sign up to be a guinea pig?

❀ ⟊ ❁

Oh, the irony! It strikes me that I've joined the same ranks as many of my clients who were stricken with a condition that medical, legal, and insurance circles debated. Claims of sick buildings, of chemical injury, of inability to work or live as they once did. I worked to prove their losses. Toxins! Now, I understand when they told me how their illnesses changed everything. I get it! Those million-dollar verdicts could never compensate them for all the anguish that forever changed their lives.

I'm glad I was able to make their lives somewhat better in securing needed funds, but there is no amount of compensation that could ever reimburse them for all the losses. Now, I would fight with all my might to help them, but my brain isn't up to that challenge.

❀ ⟊ ❁

Even the knowledge there will be minimal peace during sleep is not consoling. I used to look forward to sleeping, to not be aware of the pain, but sleep is no longer the respite it once offered. It is fitful and I'm aware of pain coursing through my body, here then there, even in an altered state.

❀ ⟊ ❁

Squish in the temples—punch in the stomach—squeeze in the esophagus. One thing's for sure … I've got the Humpty Dumpty syndrome. No one knows how to put me back together again.

My brain bounces back and forth like a ping pong ball and my head shakes from side to side. How all these symptoms have persisted is a mystery, as well as what precipitated them. I feel my nerves permeating throughout my body. Maybe this replicates Chinese water torture; yet no external forces are present. The control mechanisms are hard to locate, and even more difficult to repair.

❀ ⟊ ❁

Fatigued? How? I am totally sedentary and can't figure out how I can feel so tired, almost all the time. No energy. The constant loud buzzing and ringing in my ears is quite disturbing. I can't get rid of it. Would someone answer that phone? Whoops, it's not the phone, but my ears!

I'm also tired of being dizzy and feeling faint. The dizziness flows down to my gut. It seems my body is so unbalanced now. Perhaps that's why I'm dizzy all the time because everything in my body is out of balance.

✽ ⑃ ❋

As the brain constricts, my attitude debilitates and deteriorates. This is getting more severe every moment. Not severe enough for hospitalization or medical treatment since that hasn't seemed to work anyway, but severe enough to experience incredible pain.

The brain is floating in the shell and not being put to proper use. It feels as though I've got a meteor shower of brain waves inside. They're constantly colliding with one another with increasing force. Thump, thump, thump. My head and heart are pounding. My ears are ringing. My brain is struggling to keep things on an even keel.

✽ ⑃ ❋

Where is the successful conclusion to my story? I want this situation to be eliminated. It is difficult to think daily of sustaining my life as the seconds tick away. Pain. No purpose. No help.

Holding on becomes increasingly difficult as the symptoms escalate. No conventional test has been able to diagnose the cause nor is suggestive of a cure. Persistent feeling of riding in a roller coaster but moving only downward where my stomach is in my throat and my head remains in a vice. I can't get out of my body. I am aware of the ticking of the clock. My heart is strong, but my constitution is weak. What will become of my fate?

✽ ⑃ ❋

It seems that I'm a victim of a plague, with my body tormented from some invisible force. The worst part is that no one seems to know what has stricken me or how to help. It's been over a month since I had a stable day. I have no clue why I had a string of stable days or why I'm in a downward spiral.

I've been wanting to get out of this body for a long time, but don't know how. There is no escaping this draining feeling.

Brightness—I see sunshine on a cloudy day. Those of us facing physical adversity experience a darkness of spirit, faith, hope and trust. I for one, would like to "adjust my brightness dial" so I could always be seen as a shining star. What comes to mind is the Festival of Lights during Hannukah. It's simple to turn on a new light on the candle holder, but not so simple to light my brain's gray matter and come up with some bright ideas.

I need calm, soothing energy to assist with my healing. I desire to quell the nausea and nervousness, feelings that are persistent and pervasive. I have debilitation yet affirm potential progress. I have a strong desire to be healed yet my quality of life has deteriorated.

At this hour, I await whatever healing may become available. There is no test to measure the degree of discomfort and misery it creates. The universe has many mysteries, and although we have made many scientific discoveries, there is much left to the unknown, including what happens to people suffering without answers.

Calm the fire in the volcano—all this inflammation in my body! Stop the lava from flowing. As the earth rotates and sun rises, so does the "lava" in the body, bubble up. It's like the fire is ready to blow and spew all over my brain.

My brain has come back from its altered state and that is mostly a good thing. It still doesn't leave me with the same personality I'd like to exhibit. I often argue with Sandy when she says, "I don't know who you are anymore." Sometimes I don't know who I really am either and that is extraordinarily disconcerting.

Hold to the belief of divine intervention. Destroy feelings of distress and despair. Claim the goodness of God. Visualize wholeness and light. Focus on the soul. Know that I have the power to draw spirit into my body for the purpose of total wellbeing. I have complete faith that my angels will work wonders for me so that I can move forward with purpose and love.

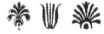

In some of those present moments of clarity, he penned some beautiful reflections of love and gratitude.

❦ ❦ ❦ ❦ ❦ ❦ ❦

Truth

For nearly two years I've been seeking an angel
by praying to heaven above.
While all this time you've been by my side;
The woman with whom I'm in love.

Why was I blind in my quest for the angel
while I lay in deep thought in my bed?
I was gripping my stomach and rubbing my chest
and taking some pills for my head.

You drove me to many appointments
for countless numbers of tests;
Like me, you suffered pain and sadness
and hardly got any rest.

I saw no less than twenty specialists
among others and such;
It was our goal to locate an answer
for which we both yearned very much.

About three dozen prescriptions
have been taken throughout these days;
I'd certainly like to cut back on these
but sadly I have no say.

God, Christ, and Holy Spirit
are beckoned to ease the pain;
Meditation and positive prayers
are offered that are never taken in vain.

God's spirit shines so brightly
all throughout the day;
I often pause and reflect on the Light
and stop for a moment to pray.

I beseech God to strengthen within me
an understanding heart;
with renewal, faith, and confidence,
I'll certainly do my part.

I open myself to receiving peace
and guidance from above;
and look forward to sharing with others
my own abundant love.

I give thanks to God
for the blessing that you truly are;
you emanate joy, love, and beauty
brighter than the brightest star.

I searched for a hidden meaning
to this lesson of life;
A search involving sorrow
and so much painful strife.

I focused on the qualities
of patience, faith, and trust;
and believing in a Godly power
was an absolute must.

With voice raised for all to know
your soul is a gift from above;
I praise the miracle that brought you here
and forever do promise my love.

Richard Strauss
December 25, 2005

221

His end-of-year reflections, drafted on his birthday a year later, offers a snapshot of his cognitive status along with a deep dive into his core values and spiritual revelations that accompanied his journey.

December 23, 2006

My Dear Daughters and Wife,

I feel sorrier for you than for myself that I am not the same Dad I was in late summer 2003, when we were whisking through the Alps, hand-clapping, yodeling, and singing along with the Sound of Music. My treatment team tells me I'll never be the same Rick. I have, however, come a long way since the epileptic-type activity witnessed by you and the writhing pain you've seen me in at the Gardens [care facility]. It's a little rationalizing, but somewhat helpful to think about the small steps to improvement. On this birthday, I pause in reflection.

Being a father is a great responsibility and a great joy. From the moment their children are born, fathers face the daily tasks of being mentors, protectors, providers, and friends. A father takes great pride in watching his children take their first steps, learn to read, and attend their first day of school. From the early days of pre-school through high school years, a father is integrally involved in other events including attending dance recitals, watching his daughter receive her National Honor Society certificate, learning to drive, and leave home to "move in" to college.

Fathers have indispensable roles to play in the lives of their children: provider, protector, nurturer, and teacher. A very caring father unconditionally loves his daughter and strives for the best for her in the future. In seeking to give his children the opportunity to succeed, fathers offer needed strength, guidance, and discipline. A father's example helps shape the character and values that his children will carry with them into adulthood and the lessons he teaches remain with them for a lifetime. By encouraging his daughters to set high standards, work hard, and make good decisions, a father shows her she can meet life's challenges.

A father's child is surrounded by love and taught the importance of respect, honesty, and integrity. Through their words, actions, and sacrifices, fathers play an important role in shaping the characters of their daughters. The time and attention that a father gives to a child is irreplaceable. There is no substitute for the involvement and commitment of a responsible father. I gave up employment security for something far more important ... your future ... and I am a much better soul for that.

When Mom and I were discussing "family," I gave no thought to the responsibilities included in the job description of a father. Nothing in college prepared me for what was to come. The "how to" books suggested general principles; however, as things came up, I took a "by the seat of my pants" approach, hoping some solution would work. There was nothing I could easily access which addressed such situations.

Fortunately, my spiritual core values helped me invoke the greatest of God's gifts—unconditional love. Along with love came caring and protection. You may be able to express a short list of other aspects but these two are paramount as to my role.

I now believe in a Divine Plan. What does that mean? Simply that each of our "ups" and few "downs" happened for a reason. I also believe that my illness was part of a plan that I co-created. On the surface, the illness sent shock waves into our family structure that had a profound ripple effect. I think now that I am back from that altered state, the lessons that we all needed to learn were achieved at least on a subconscious level, with more undoubtedly to come.

The core of my lesson was to experience a "Spiritual Awakening" that, by analogy, was like the scene in ET when he appeared to be dying; you saw the flowers regenerate while simultaneously ET came back to life and eventually found his way "home." This is a clear example of a major shift in consciousness.

I know that I'm not always the easiest person in the world to get along with now. There are times when I'm moody. Not that I didn't get moody before, but now the emotionality is partly blamed on brain damage. I'm working on that with Dr. D in therapy and neuro-biofeedback and will be taking a meditation class after the first of the year.

It is my belief that I have come back stronger and more devoted than ever. I have completed much of that spiritual shift to which I referred and think I am a better person for it. I do not expect perfection, but I do expect better results as I focus on a number of universal laws, especially the Law of Attraction. I see good coming to me now as I believe in the ample supply of resources available to me in the universe and consciously focus on ways of bringing those resources to me so I may use them to fit my individual needs. I am also listening harder and paying more attention to cues that may come to me so I can take appropriate action.

I am also speaking my truth more than ever and speaking from the heart. I know I often display a weird and wacky persona, but deep down I often have an important message to share to fulfill my mission—my passion of helping another person. What the person does with the message is for them to reflect upon and process.

My mother, your dear Nana, was the Queen of Analogies and I know I inherited that trait as I often impart a message using an "out of the box," sometimes funny comparison. That ability to crystallize by analogy as always been one of my touchstones, and believe it or not, it often works. That fact that I succeeded for 20 years in my own business is a testament to that.

I have usually spoken my truth from the heart and will always "be straight" with you while concurrently respecting your individual set of values. I thank the Holy Spirit for bringing you into my life. That even has enriched my life forever.

I am proud and blessed to be your daddy and husband.

I love you dearly. Happy holidays. As a matter of fact, happy days thereafter as well.

Rick

Dear God,

My spirituality has grown through this process. I have become somewhat separated from my wife. As I wrote some years ago:

> I don't know where I'm going.
> But I know where I have been and
> When I get there, I'll know that I am.

Well, that's not exact, but close enough as I am aware my life is but a series of fleeting moments. I am not able to relive the joys or pains of the past. I cannot foresee with authority the future. All I can do is embrace my divinity and live the best life for me possible in the eternity of the nowness.

Richard
December 31, 2006

Such insights into his soul's journey. Less than a month later, Rick moved out and was living alone, unsupervised. As his brain became more inflamed in the ensuing months, his writings to us became correspondingly fiery and abusive. Gratefully, this phase stopped when he was hospitalized. After that, Rick never wrote again but thankfully, returned over time to express his loving, compassionate nature.

His death in April 2016 was the end of our story together, but his legacy continues as I now step forward as if by assignment—by sharing our journey and the revelations from it, in service to other weary spirits who may be facing their own challenging conditions.

Life doesn't do anything to you, it just reveals your spirit.
Author unknown

Appendices

Appendix A
Recognizing Neurotoxicity

This article is written by a neurotoxic forensic expert witness whose testimony is often decisive in legal cases with expertise of the toxic substance's effects on nervous system function (neurobehavioral toxicity, neurotoxicology). It validates the impact of toxicity upon brain injury relative to mood, behavior and other symptoms and the difficulties doctors have in proper evaluation.

***

A person's ability to think, perceive, control emotions, plan, and manage his or her life can diminish drastically without anything being visible to a radiologist or neurologist on an MRI or a CT scan.

Dr. Raymond Singer

Neurotoxicity—poisoning of the brain and nervous system—is a well-documented effect of exposure to many widely used chemicals, yet doctors (and lawyers) often fail to recognize it. Chemically injured clients often report a confusing array of symptoms, with no medical diagnosis. The symptoms may seem vague and unconnected, leading you to wonder, "Could these symptoms really be caused by a chemical exposure?"

A person who has suffered a serious chemical injury is likely to have sustained considerable damage to his or her brain and nervous system.

Neurotoxicity can be documented, but perhaps not in the way you might think. A person's ability to think, perceive, control emotions, plan, and manage his or her life can diminish drastically without anything being visible to a radiologist or neurologist on an MRI or a CT scan.

The most reliable and widely accepted way to assess actual brain function is through neuropsychological evaluation. (This is true for head-injury patients and those suffering from dementia, as well as those affected by exposure to toxic chemicals.)

Researchers have noted that imaging techniques are often of little value in evaluating neurotoxicity. In our and others' experience, imaging techniques can occasionally pick up abnormalities caused by neurotoxicity and may be helpful for forensic purposes, but they are not cost-beneficial for routine screening.

Neuropsychological testing tends to be more sensitive to brain injury than CT and routine MRI scans, which provide only a static and relatively gross view of neural structure. In 1 study of 6 head-injury cases, CT and/or MRI scans yielded little or no evidence of neuropathology as detected by neuropsychological testing. Positron emission tomography (PET) scans, however, corroborated the impaired function. PET and SPECT (single photon emission computed tomography) scans offer a more dynamic look at brain structure, but both of these tests still need interpretation as to the cause of the abnormality (which could be benign). Each of these tests offer different diagnostic capabilities which are described below.

Common Symptoms

What do chronic pain, anxiety, neurological problems, confusion, psychiatric symptoms, and cognitive declines have in common? They can all result from neurotoxic chemical exposure.

Symptoms of neurotoxicity include memory and concentration problems; confusion; multiple sclerosis or MS-type symptoms; impaired control of the limbs, bladder, or bowels; headaches or migraines; sleep disorders, including sleep apnea; eye problems that are neurological in origin; balance and hearing problems; muscle weakness; anxiety or panic attacks; depression; and other psychiatric or neurological symptoms.

Other symptoms that could be caused by chemical injury include multi-organ system malfunction; lower or upper respiratory problems, such as chronic sinus problems; multiple chemical sensitivity (MCS); liver or kidney problems; and fibromyalgia or other pain disorders.

Along with nervous system dysfunction, the temporal association of any of these conditions with toxic chemical exposure tends to support the theory that the overall cause of the client's injuries is a toxic insult to the body.

The patient with "too many" symptoms can get a diagnosis of "somatic disorder"—that is, having physical symptoms caused by psychological conditions. This misdiagnosis says that psychological problems are the underlying cause of the illness.

It is not unusual for patients suffering from neurotoxicity to be misdiagnosed as having psychological problems because of their depression and anxiety levels, the sheer number of their symptoms, and their belief that chemicals made them ill.

Source: "Recognizing Neurotoxicity" by Raymond Singer and Dana Darby Johnson, *Trial,* March 2006, 62. Reprinted with permission of the Association of Trial Lawyers of America. Additional information especially relevant to legal cases is available from: http://neurotox.com/project/recognizing-neurotoxicity.

Distinctive Differences in Diagnostic Scans

CT: (computed tomography uses X-rays to create detailed pictures of organs, bones, and other tissues. The data can be assembled to form 3D images which can reveal abnormalities in both bone and soft tissues including bleeding in the brain (hemorrhage), blood clots (hematomas), bruised brain tissue (contusions), and brain tissue swelling.

MRI (magnetic resonance imaging) also creates detailed pictures using radio waves and a powerful magnet, providing images of internal organs and tissues showing the difference between normal and diseased tissue. MRIs can detect diseases more reliably than via a CT scan with some cancers or tissues, i.e. metastases to the bone and brain. It can also help to detect traumatic brain injury, developmental anomalies, multiple sclerosis, stroke, dementia, infection, and the causes of headache.

PET: Positron emission tomography is nuclear imaging which uses small amounts of radioactive materials called radiotracers, a special camera, and a computer to evaluate organ and tissue functions on a cellular level. PET scans have capabilities that often can detect abnormalities in organs and tissues before other diagnostic imaging. It is used to diagnose cancer, heart, brain disease and other conditions. A combination PET-CT scan produces 3D images for a more accurate diagnosis.[1]

Brain SPECT: (single photon emission computed tomography) is a state-of-the-art brain mapping tool, using nuclear medicine that is proven to reliably evaluate blood flow and brain activity. This assists in the evaluation of brain function abnormalities including dementia, stroke, head injury, seizures, tumors, brain inflammation, Lyme disease, chemical exposure, depression, and other disorders.[2]

Volumetric MRI: An additional diagnostic tool of the traditional MRI. It segments and measures the volumes of various brain structures and compares them to norms, providing more visual and quantitative information useful in assessments.

Appendix B
The Ticking Time Bomb of Lyme

The conclusion is the number of people with chronic Lyme disease likely ranges between 1 and 3 million, and the annual cost—for chronic Lyme disease alone—may top $75 billion a year.[1]

LymeDisease.org

Lyme disease is indeed a ticking time bomb because it is notoriously difficult to diagnose. While there are many species of Lyme, only a handful of strains are detectable with current technology, so health professionals might erroneously rule out Lyme disease. Yet, it may be the root cause of a patient's illness. The traditional lab tests for Lyme yield false negative results for an estimated 20-30% of patients who are infected. There are several reasons for this, according to the website, LymeDisease.org, which advocates nationally for quality accessible healthcare: the immune system may be suppressed and there may not have been enough time for antibodies to develop, or the person may be infected with a strain the test doesn't measure.

The challenges associated with a Lyme diagnosis is further compounded by significant controversies in science, medicine, and public policy regarding the disease itself. Together, these obstacles make it difficult for patients to be properly diagnosed and receive treatment. An infected person may not even realize that they were infected since the distinctive "bulls-eye" rash doesn't even appear in 25-50% of the cases.[2] Not receiving proper treatment can be dangerous for all the complications Lyme disease creates.

Neurotoxins are released by the spirochetes associated with Lyme disease often with co-infections with other tick-borne organisms, including *Babesia, Bartonella* and others. The infections caused by them release their poisons, circulating throughout the body, clinging to the brain, nerves, glands, organs, and other tissues, saturating them with this toxicity.

If Lyme disease is properly diagnosed, a course of antibiotics is typically given, but if lab tests cannot confirm Lyme, then the infected person may not be given antibiotics. And, if they're genetically poor detoxifiers, they will likely experience post-Lyme symptoms, leading to a lifetime of misery. The CRBAI estimates that about 25% of the population are genetically poor detoxifiers, which can lead to multiple debilitating issues associated with chronic Lyme disease.

It's not uncommon for Lyme patients to be misdiagnosed and labeled with other debilitating health issues, such as chronic fatigue syndrome, fibromyalgia, multiple sclerosis, autoimmune diseases, and various psychiatric illnesses.

Many symptoms of Lyme disease and other neurotoxin diseases include loss of enthusiasm, disorganization, or lack of planning and executive skills, among many others. These poisons diminish the release and the availability of neurotransmitters, which can lead to brain process issues including: focus, movement, balance and coordination problems, stiffness, rigidity, joint and muscle pain, and others.

The longer one is ill with Lyme, the more neurotoxic poison is present in the body, which challenges full recovery. When Lyme disease affects the brain, it is referred to as Lyme neuroborreliosis or Lyme encephalopathy, which can mimic virtually any type of encephalopathy.

Based on the most recent insurance records, the Centers for Disease Control and Prevention suggest that approximately 476,000 Americans are diagnosed and treated for Lyme disease annually. Lyme Disease is placing a large burden on the health care system, demonstrating the need for more effective prevention and diagnostic measures.[3]

Appendix C
The Forbidden Foods on an Amylose-Free Diet

Patients suffering from mold illness should take caution consuming foods containing amylose. Amylose is known as the "starchy, non-sticky starch" in cooking. Typically, amylose offers many benefits. However, for patients stricken with Chronic Inflammatory Response Syndrome (CIRS) it has the potential to worsen conditions.

According to Pattie Rose MSN, a board-certified functional nurse practitioner, "The No Amylose Diet will help to bring down elevated MMP9 levels which are seen in Chronic Inflammatory Response Syndrome (CIRS) and to help prevent chronic diseases as a result of obesity. Diets high in these foods can also contribute to Candida overgrowth in the gut causing many of the same symptoms of mold sickness like irritability, anxiety, skin rashes, brain fog, and difficulty losing weight. Sugar is fungi's favorite snack. Starve the fungus right out of your body."[1]

Foods to avoid: This is a general list below. Avoid foods with high amylose and sugar. For more detailed information of dietary choices, visit www.moldfreemenu.com.

- Roots and tubers, including all potatoes—white, sweet, yams etc., beets, peanuts, carrots, jicama, parsnip, turnip, taro, and other vegetables that grow underground. The exception here is onions and garlic.
- Fruits.
  - Bananas. The Shoemaker website states this is "the only forbidden fruit," however other high sugar fruits can cause blood sugar spikes like these high glycemic fruits:
    - Pineapple
    - Mango
    - Melons
    - Oranges
    - Grapes

All foods with added sugar, sucrose, corn syrup, or maltodextrin are strictly forbidden. Table sugar and all other simple, fast-releasing sugars, such as fructose, lactose, maltose, glucose, mannitol, and sorbitol. This includes honey and natural syrup type products, such as maple syrup and molasses. Generally, all candies, sweets, cakes, cookies, soft drinks (diet too), and baked goods, unless they are made ONLY from approved foods above. Whole leaf stevia concentrate may be used in moderation (though it does have some side effects) *Over time, high levels of blood sugar may lead to various chronic diseases like Type 2 diabetes.*

- Wheat

- Rye

- Barley

- Oats

- Tapioca

- Cornstarch

- Rice (all kinds) Dr. Shoemaker from Survivingmold.com does not allow rice.

- Potatoes—all of them. Even sweet potatoes and yams.

- Condiments: vinegar and foods containing vinegar: mayonnaise, pickles, soy sauce, mustard, relishes. They contain sugar and or vinegar (fermented). You can make some on your own from fresh ingredients and omit the forbidden foods.

- All processed foods. Canned, boxed, bottled, cured, aged, etc. They are much more likely to contain added sugar, chemicals, and mycotoxins. Foods like baked beans, soups, commercial sauces, soft drinks, fruit juices, condiments, sauces, ready-made meals, breakfast cereals, candy, ice cream, frozen meals, smoked meats: sausages, hot dogs, corned beef, pastrami, smoked fish, ham, and bacon are a few examples.

- All trans fats are highly inflammatory and strictly forbidden.

- Palm oil.

- Generic vegetable oil.

As noted on their website: "The information we provide at Moldfreemenu. com intends to provide data that clarifies how a healthy diet is part of healing from biotoxin illness. The information does not intend to replace consultation with a qualified medical professional. Specific medical advice, including diagnosis and treatment are not available from MFM. This diet does not cure mold illness, but does help reduce inflammation (provided you avoid all items your body reacts to)—thus reducing symptoms triggered by inflammation."[2]

For recipes and menu ideas visit www.moldfreemenu.com.

Appendix D
Common Symptoms of Lewy Body Dementia

Each person with LBD is different in terms of which symptoms they have in the beginning. The most common symptoms include changes in thinking, behavior, movement, and sleep.

- **Dementia** refers to a significant decline in thinking ability. With LBD it affects memory, decision making, problem solving, planning, and abstract or analytical thinking.

- **Cognitive fluctuations** involve unpredictable changes in concentration, alertness, or attention.

- **Parkinson's-like symptoms** include slowness of movement, rigidity or stiffness, shuffling gait, tremors, and balance problems.

- **Behavioral changes** include hallucinations, delusions, or changes in mood.

  - **Hallucinations** are seeing or hearing things that are not really present and can occur in other senses like hearing, touch and smell. If the hallucinations are not disruptive, they may not need to be treated. However, if they are frightening or create challenging behavioral changes, your physician may recommend treatment.

  - **Delusions** (false beliefs) and paranoia (unwarranted suspicions) can occur, sometimes alone or in response to threatening hallucinations.

  - **Changes in mood**, including depression, anxiety, and apathy, are extremely common in LBD and may significantly affect your quality of life.

- **Sleep disorders** include REM sleep behavior disorder (RBD), excessive daytime sleepiness, temporary loss of consciousness with difficulties wakening, insomnia, and restless leg syndrome. These sleep problems can be subtle and hard to diagnose. RBD involves acting out dreams and may result in injuries from hitting bed partners or falling out of bed. Symptoms of RBD may appear years before any of the other symptoms of LBD.

- **Autonomic symptoms** are common in LBD. The autonomic nervous system controls many involuntary functions. Problems with temperature and blood pressure regulation can occur, as well as constipation, urinary incontinence, unexplained blackouts or transient loss of consciousness, and sexual dysfunction. Low blood pressure can cause dizziness and fainting when a person stands from a sitting or lying position too quickly.

Note: LBDA developed a useful checklist to help physicians and their patients identify key LBD symptoms used to make a diagnosis.

Source: Lewy Body Dementia Association[1]

Appendix E
Differences between Alzheimer's Disease and Lewy body Dementia

Alzheimer's disease symptoms include a progressive loss of recent memory; problems with language, calculation, abstract thinking, and judgment; depression or anxiety; personality and behavioral changes; and disorientation to time and place. LBD is frequently misdiagnosed as Alzheimer's disease, especially in the early stage. Over time, changes in movement, hallucinations or RBD can help distinguish LBD from Alzheimer's disease.

Lewy body dementia (LBD) is an umbrella term for a form of dementia that has three common presentations.

- *Some individuals will start out with a change in thinking* that may resemble Alzheimer's disease, but over time two or more distinctive features become apparent leading to the diagnosis of '*dementia with Lewy bodies*' (DLB). Symptoms that differentiate it from Alzheimer's include unpredictable levels of cognitive ability, attention or alertness, changes in walking or movement, visual hallucinations, a sleep disorder called REM sleep behavior disorder, in which people physically act out their dreams, and severe sensitivity to medications for hallucinations. In some cases, the sleep disorder can precede the dementia and other symptoms of LBD by decades.

- *Others will start out with a movement disorder* leading to the diagnosis of Parkinson's disease and later develop dementia and other symptoms common in DLB.

- Lastly, *a small group will first present with neuropsychiatric symptoms*, which can include hallucinations, behavioral problems, and difficulty with complex mental activities, leading to an initial diagnosis of DLB.

Regardless of the initial symptom, over time all three presentations of LBD will develop very similar cognitive, physical, sleep and behavioral features, all caused by the presence of Lewy bodies throughout the brain.

Source: Lewy Body Dementia Association[1]

Appendix F
Functional Evaluation for Type 3 (Toxic) Alzheimer's Disease

As referenced earlier in the posthumous postscript section of the story of our journey, Rick's lab results, characteristics, biomarkers, and symptoms are in alignment with Dr. Bredesen's research, linking biotoxins and other toxic compounds now underlying a newly defined type of AD. This research also reinforces the crucial value of functional evaluation with its precise testing pinpointing underlying issues and the imbalances created from them. It is precision testing of a patient's biochemistry, offering insights into therapies, rather than based on reviewing the symptoms to make a diagnosis or assign a code.

Posthumous Proof: Comparing Rick's labs which had been collected 11 years earlier during consultations with Dr. Ritchie Shoemaker to those of Dr. Bredesen's team, identifying characteristics of Alzheimer's Type 3 (toxic-related), validated the organic nature of his illness, linked to its toxic roots. Previously, these had been dismissed or discredited by nearly all of Rick's mainstream medical doctors while we were searching for answers. As groundbreaking research, it was still too early for this to have become mainstream knowledge.

Dr. Bredesen's team of peer-reviewed research provided legitimacy to Rick's case, long denied by conventional practitioners consulting with us. Bredesen's research was in alignment with Rick's lab work almost a dozen years earlier and reflected the same characteristics of his illness. Yet, we had not encountered any allopathic physician willing to explore its connections to toxicity.

It did not matter to me what the condition was called, if it accurately described the manifestation of all the symptoms, behaviors, and the inflammation underlying them all. However, what is important for readers to recognize is that toxicity was at the root of Rick's illness. Especially for the benefit of others seeking answers—if patients are exhibiting neurological symptoms that it is imperative they be properly evaluated for toxic exposures. If present, it is then vital that the correct therapies are administered for treatment and detoxification.

(See chapters 19 and 20 for more background.)

Type 3 Alzheimer's disease: Here is the chart illustrating how Rick's test results and characteristics of his illness align with Dr. Bredesen's research.

Source:
Characteristics of type 3 Alzheimer's disease (from Bredesen, Aging, 2016. 3)[1]

Characteristic	Comment
Symptoms begin before age 65.	Symptoms often begin in the fifties or late forties.
Usually ApoE4.	Typically ApoE3/3.
No family history, or family history with symptoms Beginning only at ages much older than the patient's.	The few with positive family histories are often those with ApoE4.
Symptoms often occur around the time of menopause or andropause.	Hormone status appears to be intimately related to type 3 Alzheimer's disease.
Depression precedes or accompanies the cognitive decline.	Depression is often associated with HPA axis (hypothalamic-pituitary-adrenal) hormonal dysfunction.
Headache is an early symptom, and sometimes the first.	Headache is a common feature in association with toxin exposure.
Memory consolidation is neither the initial nor the dominant symptom.	Typical symptoms include executive function deficits (planning, problem solving, organizing, focusing), Inability to manipulate numbers/ perform calculations, trouble speaking or loss of speech, problems with visual perception, or problems with learned programs such as dressing.
Precipitation or exacerbation by great stress (e.g. loss of employment, divorce, family change) and sleep loss.	The degree of dysfunction is also markedly affected by stress and sleep loss.
Exposure to mycotoxins or metals (e.g. inorganic mercury via amalgams or organic mercury via fish) or both.	Exposures can be evaluated by blood and urine tests.
Diagnosis of CIRS (chronic inflam-matory response syndrome) with cognitive decline.	Cognitive decline is common with CIRS.
Imaging suggest brain changes not seen in most cases of Alzheimer's.	FDG-PET may show frontal as well as tempo-roparietal reductions in glucose utilization, even early in the course of the illness; MRI may show generalized shrinkage in the cerebral cortex and cerebellum, especially with mild FLAIR (fluid-at-tenuated inversion recovery) hyperintensity.
Low serum triglycerides or low ratio of triglycerides to total cholesterol.	Triglycerides are often in the 50's.
Low serum zinc (<75mcg/dl) or RBC zinc, or ratio of copper to zinc >1.3	Copper to zinc ratio should be 1.0, and values >1.3 are associated with cognitive decline.
HPA axis dysfunction, with low pregnenolone, DHEA-S and/or AM cortisol.	Hormonal abnormalities are common in this type of Alzheimer's disease.
High serum C4a, TGF-ß1 or MMp9; or low serum MSH (melanocyte-stimulating hormone.)	These tests indicate exposure to biotoxins such as mycotoxins.
HLA-DR/DQ associated with multiple biot6oxin sensitivities or pathogen-specific sensitivity.	This generic test indicates that you are particularly sensitive to biotoxins, and is positive in about 25 percent of people.

The biomarker Matrix Metallopeptidase 9 (MMP9) is an enzyme that breaks down cell membranes in the vessel walls, delivering inflammatory elements from the blood affecting brain, muscle, lung, peripheral nerves, and joints. In CIRS patients, the inflammatory cytokines, activate white blood cells to release MMP9 into the bloodstream causing widespread inflammation.

The C3a and C4a blood serum measurements are valuable in the evaluation of the immune system's ability to turn itself off. Conventional practitioners routinely measure inflammation with the C-reactive protein or erythrocyte sedimentation rate (or "sed rate"). However, these lab tests are not an accurate diagnostic tool of inflammation for biotoxic patients. So, without these specialized biomarkers, healthcare practitioners are unable to precisely assess the inflammatory nature of the patient's condition.

Glossary

AD: acronym for Alzheimer's Disease.

Allele: one of two or more versions of a gene; we inherit two alleles for each gene, one from each parent.

Amylose: a complex plant starch in a group of carbohydrates that isn't well-digested or absorbed in the small intestine and prevents the rapid rise of blood sugar after a meal. Low-amylose diets are advised for those being treated for biotoxin illnesses.

APOE: a gene that affects the likelihood for developing Alzheimer's disease by influencing the number of harmful plaques in the brain. The e4 version of the APOE gene increases an individual's risk for developing late-onset Alzheimer disease. APOE is responsible for removing plaques from the brain, believed to be one of the primary causes of Alzheimer's.

Autoimmune disorder: refers to dysregulation of the immune system, causing immune cells to attack the body. Autoimmune responses can affect any and many parts of the body.

Autophagy: the process of cleaning out damaged cells in order to regenerate newer, healthier cells.

Biomarker: a test that reflects biological activity of an illness. Some are static, such as a genetic marker. Others are dynamic and change with disease activity.

Biotoxin illness: chronic inflammatory condition, which creates a cascade of symptoms in those who are genetically susceptible and unable to clear exposures from biologically produced neurotoxins (known as biotoxins and inflammagens).

Biotoxin Pathway: characterizes a complex pattern of biochemical reactions in genetically-prone people to bio toxic exposures and imbalances created by the continuing, unregulated production of cytokines.

Bipolar disorder: is a mental health condition that causes extreme mood swings with characteristic emotional highs (mania) and lows (depression).

Blood brain barrier (BBB): the brain's protective barrier that allows essential nutrients to cross into the brain, yet prevents toxins and other harmful particles from crossing over.

Body burden: term used to describe the total accumulation of toxins in your body.

BPA (bisphenol A): an industrial chemical used to make certain plastics and epoxy resins.

Chelation: a form of therapy for removing heavy metals, such as mercury or lead from the blood. It's one of the standard treatments for many types of metals poisoning.

Chronic Inflammatory Response Syndrome (CIRS): a multi-symptom, multi-system condition triggered by inhaling, ingesting, or transdermally introducing biotoxins and inflammagens, produced by micro-organisms, such as mold and bacteria, into the body. It is a progressive illness that can affect virtually any organ system and become debilitating if left untreated.

Closed kinetic chain exercises: Also known as closed chain exercises, these are physical exercises performed where the hand (for arm movement) or foot (for leg movement) is fixed in space and cannot move.

Cognoscopy: is a comprehensive evaluation using a combination of laboratory and cognitive testing that identify the contributors to cognitive decline or risk for decline.

Complement system: part of the immune system that critically important to protect against infection.

Cortisol: known as the stress hormone because of its role in the body's stress response. High cortisol levels are detrimental and can cause many unwanted symptoms.

Cytokines: molecules that allow your cells to communicate with one another and are crucial for healthy immune system function. They're released by one cell to regulate the function of another cell.

Dementogens: A name given to categories of toxins that can lead to dementia.

Detoxification: the metabolic process by which toxins are changed into less toxic or more readily excretable substances. It is widely used in functional and integrative practices, based on the principle that illnesses are caused by the accumulation of toxic substances (toxins) in the body. Eliminating existing toxins and avoiding new toxins are essential parts of the healing process.

DLB: acronym for Dementia with Lewy bodies.

DNA methylation: one of several epigenetic mechanisms that cells use to control gene expression. Methylation is important for proper functioning of many processes, including energy production, heavy-metal detoxification, and hormone balance, as well as cardiovascular, immune, and nervous system activity.

DSM (*Diagnostic and Statistical Manual of Mental Disorders*): the principal authority for psychiatric diagnoses in the United States. Treatment recommendations, as well as payment by healthcare providers, are often determined by DSM classifications.

Dysbiosis: an unhealthy change in the body's microbial communities, often noted in the gastrointestinal tract and associated with health problems and diseases.

EDTA: a chemical that binds and holds on to (chelates) minerals and metals, such as chromium, iron, lead, mercury, copper, aluminum, nickel, zinc, calcium, cobalt, manganese, and magnesium.

EMF (Electromagnetic Field): grouped into two types of EMF exposures: 1) non-ionizing, low-level radiation from appliances such as microwave ovens, cellphones, Wi-Fi routers, Smart meters, power lines, and MRIs, and 2) ionizing radiation emitted from ultraviolet light and X-rays. There's disagreement among scientists regarding the safety of EMFs.

Encephalopathy: a general term describing a disease that affects the function or structure of the brain. The main symptom associated with encephalopathy is an altered mental state.

Endocrine disrupters: found in many products, including some plastic bottles and containers, liners of metal food cans, detergents, flame retardants, food, toys, cosmetics, and pesticides. These interfere with different endocrine glands, such as the thyroid, ovaries, testes, and adrenal glands and the hormones produced by them.

Epigenetics: the study of how your behaviors and environment can cause changes affecting the expression of your genes. It's a rapidly growing area of science that explores the processes that help influence whether individual genes are turned on or off.

Functional medicine: a systems biology-based approach that focuses on identifying and addressing the root cause of disease. This model of care offers a patient-centered approach to chronic disease management by exploring the root causes of a person's symptoms, such as poor nutrition, stress, toxins, allergens, genetics, and the microbiome.

Genetic susceptibility: a predetermined group of immune-response genes represented by HLA DR.

Genotype: refers to a person's genetic makeup and specific DNA sequence.

GI: acronym for gastrointestinal.

Glutathione: an antioxidant produced in cells. Glutathione levels in the body may be reduced by several factors, including poor nutrition, environmental toxins, and stress. Levels of this important nutrient decline with age.

GMO (genetically modified organism): a living being, e.g., an animal, plant, or microbe whose DNA has been altered using genetic engineering techniques.

Heavy metals: dense metals, such as lead, mercury, chromium, copper, and others that are usually toxic at low concentrations.

HLA DR: an indicator of groups of immune-response genes. Genetic testing determines whether you are genetically unable to properly detect and eliminate biotoxins from toxic agents via the immune system. An estimated 25% of the population who carry the HLA-DRBQ gene are unable to make antibodies needed to deactivate and remove mold toxins.

Homeopathy: a medical system based on the belief that the body can cure itself. Practitioners use tiny amounts of natural substances, like plants and minerals, to stimulate the healing process.

Inflammagens: multiple agents, such as toxins, that cause inflammatory responses.

Inflammation: a response triggered by damage to living tissues. Chronic inflammation occurs when this response lingers long-term, causing the body to be in a constant state of alert with negative impact.

Intermittent fasting: an eating pattern that cycles between periods of fasting and only eating during a specific time.

Ketones: water-soluble energy molecules made by the mitochondria in the liver from dietary or stored fats, and used as an alternative fuel to glucose.

Ketosis: when the body burns stored fat for energy instead of blood sugar.

LBD: acronym for Lewy body dementia.

Leaky brain: a term used to describe a dysfunction of the blood brain barrier (BBB) which can cause the tight junctions to become more permeable. This allows substances, including toxins, to cross over into the brain, causing brain inflammation.

Leaky gut syndrome (LGS): a digestive condition affecting the lining of the intestines. This syndrome creates gaps in the intestinal walls, allowing bacteria and other toxins to pass into the bloodstream. Scientific evidence suggests it may contribute to a range of medical conditions.

Lyme disease: an infectious and biotoxin illness caused by the spirochete, *Borrelia burgdorferi,* following a tick bite by an infected organism.

MARCoNS (multiple antibiotic-resistant coagulase negative coloniza-tion staphylococci): a colonization of germs which can occur in people with MSH deficiencies.

Methylation: (see DNA methylation).

Microbiome: the collection of all microbes, such as bacteria, fungi, viruses, and their genes, that naturally live on our bodies and inside us. A healthy microbiome contributes to health and wellness.

MMP9 (matrix metalloproteinases): a marker of inflammation; a high reading is an indicator of toxins and cytokines. It is especially adept at delivering inflammatory elements out of blood vessels and placing them where they don't belong, such as in the brain, nerves, lungs, muscles, and joints.

MMSE (Mini Mental State Examination): is a 30-point questionnaire used traditionally in clinical settings to measure cognitive impairment. It is a standard screening tool for dementia.

MSH (melanocyte stimulating hormone): regulates many functions and controls many immune responses. In biotoxin patients, a cascade of symptoms appears when MSH is disrupted.

MTHFR (*methylenetetrahydrofolate reductase*): a key enzyme, which if mutated, can interfere with the body's ability to perform normally in countless, critical functions. A genetic mutation may lead to high levels of homocysteine in the blood and low levels of folate and other vitamins.

Mycotoxicosis: an acute and chronic toxic disease caused by mycotoxins.

Mycotoxin: a naturally occurring toxin produced by molds and fungi. It can cause a variety of adverse health effects.

Neuropathy: a term that refers to malfunctions of the nerves which can be damaged from injury or disease.

Neuropsychological evaluation: an assessment involving an interview and the administration of tests of how an individual's brain functions, yielding information about the structural and functional integrity of the brain.

Neurotoxicity: refers to damage related to the brain or peripheral nervous system caused by exposure to natural or man-made toxic substances (neuro-toxicants), altering the normal activity of the nervous system.

Nutrigenomics (also known as nutritional genomics): defined as the relationship between nutrients, diet, and gene expression.

PBDE (polybrominated diphenyl ethers): a class of fire-retardant chemicals.

PD: acronym for Parkinson's disease, a neurodegenerative disorder.

Phthalates: a class of chemicals commonly used as plasticizers, which are additives that improve the flexibility of plastics.

Phytonutrients: natural chemicals or compounds produced by plants, which have antioxidant and anti-inflammatory properties that help support a healthy human body.

Post-Lyme Syndrome: a collection of symptoms and abnormalities that persist in a patient with Lyme disease after treatment with antibiotics. It is often experienced in patients with certain genetics that compromise their ability to easily recover.

RBD: acronym for rapid eye movement sleep behavior disorder, which is associated with some neurological diseases.

Small Intestinal Bacterial Overgrowth (SIBO): this occurs when there is an abnormal increase in the overall bacterial population in the small intestine, especially bacteria not generally found in that part of the digestive tract.

Sick Building Syndrome (SBS): also termed environmental illness, SBS is acquired from working in buildings with poor quality air related to mold, or other indoor pollutants, e.g., formaldehyde fumes, or from water-damaged buildings. It covers a range of symptoms for those who spend time in a building with poor air quality.

Sulfation: this is part of the process critical to the body's ability to remove toxins through methylation.

TNF (tumor necrosis factor alpha): this is one of the cytokines that increases inflammation. Post-Lyme Syndrome patients often have elevated levels; it is rarely elevated in mold patients.

Vagus nerve (also known as the 10th cranial nerve): a very long nerve originating in the brain stem and extending down through the neck and into the chest and abdomen. It is the key player in the autonomic nervous system which regulates bodily functions.

VCS test (Visual Contrast Sensitivity test): a screening that indicates a distinctive group of deficits in biotoxin illness patients. It measures a person's ability to see details at low contrast levels and is useful for identifying impairments in neurological function.

VEGF (vascular endothelial growth factor): supports the delivery of oxygen. Low VEGF levels is common in biotoxic patients, which means oxygen delivery is compromised.

Acknowledgments

My intention for this book was to share the experience of my husband's debilitating, neurological disorder and what contributed to it, while also sharing insights that might prove valuable for others traveling a similar path. I want to thank the many who played important roles throughout our journey, others who offered their wisdom for enlightening content, and others for their creativity in assembling it all into this book.

I have a heart full of gratitude for Ritchie Shoemaker, MD, whose passionate research regarding the impact of biotoxins upon health was a decisive turning point for Rick, as well as the tens of thousands whose health destinies have been transformed from his wisdom. With his recognition that biotoxin-induced illnesses would become one of the most important medical topics in the 21st century, he has transformed countless health destinies with his precision diagnostics and treatments.

So have other doctors and researchers with their quest for revealing critical connections and therapies to recover patient health. That is especially true for those whose illnesses are linked to toxicity and other underlying issues and especially challenging to treat. Among them are Dale Bredesen, MD, an internationally acclaimed expert in the mechanisms of neurodegenerative diseases; David Perlmutter, MD, renowned neurologist, and Neil Nathan, MD, author of his enlightening book, *Toxic*, along with other innovative medical pioneers. They have enlightened us with groundbreaking research, helping forge brighter health destinies for conditions once considered irreversible. Without such trailblazing spirits, far too many would be stuck with hopeless diagnoses and suffer needlessly. I applaud their curiosity to explore the deeper realms of science, extract such wisdom, and bring it forth in service to humanity.

There are several integrative practitioners for whose wisdom and guidance I am especially appreciative. I have previously mentioned my fortunate connection with Dan Watts, MD, the medical reviewer and contributor for this book, whose personal battle with mold illness offered invaluable insights. His expertise was indispensable for this book's content and for my personal wellness. Special thanks to Tamy Califano for all your assistance, coordination, decoding, and cheerful countenance through it all!

With Dr. Rebecca Acosta's expertise of the complex methylation pathway, I am grateful for the guidance of Nelsa Andersson Ciapponi, MD, ABIHM, a functional practitioner at Optimal Health Medicine Center in Charlotte, NC. Her insights enriched the importance of patient education.

I wish to thank Felix Liao, DDS, of Whole Health Dental Center in Falls, Church, Virginia, and Dick Chapman, DDS of Florida Integrative Dentistry, Sarasota, Florida, for providing such in-depth information regarding the defining differences of biological dentistry and its connections to whole health.

I am most fortunate to have the dearest of friends, Reverend Lowell Smith, who offered such guidance and support throughout all the years of Rick's illness. You provided such insights that uplifted my spirits and enabled me to find peace in the most turbulent times.

I am immensely grateful to our daughters, Stephanie and Stacy, for meeting all the complexities we faced as a family while suspended in a world without answers; and to my sister, Connie DeVries and brother, Art Conrad.

With a heart full of gratitude to Larry for encouraging me to write this book and for the innumerable ways you supported Rick and our family through the challenges that dementia creates for the patient and the caregiver.

I also wish to acknowledge the network of other family and friends whose loving support and guidance during this journey lifted my spirits; their impact is immeasurable in my heart. Linda O'Dean, Cindi Callanan, Lynn Chambers, Brenda and Bob Root, David and Hollye Doane, Deborah Ross, Dottie McKee, Claudia Adams, Reverend Sandra Butler, Reverend Donna Johnson, Reverend Jane St. John, Rick and Anita Hartley, Pete and Maureen Clifford, Nina Gibson, Diana Ott Wright, Carolyn Lygo, Dottie Moore, and countless others who sustained me with their kindnesses, wisdom, and prayers. They were lifelines for my heart as reflected on a plaque received during the journey: "A friend knows the song in your heart and can sing it back to you when you've forgotten the words."

Getting a book into print requires the creative energy of many, including editors Ken Walker, Deborah Ross, and Vivie Bishop. I am grateful for the creative flair of Victoria Dolci and designers Wardell and Rosi Parker of Syzygy Media. Much appreciation to Jennifer Abernethy of Socially Delivered for your marketing genius in reaching important audiences who are especially interested in this work.

This book is a compilation of wisdom gleaned from doctors, researchers, wellness professionals and others who are transforming paradigms for people to enjoy vibrant health and robust destinies. Indeed, the wellness and wellbeing of humanity is indebted to your relentless pursuit of knowledge and health solutions.

With boundless gratitude to you all!

Notes

Why I Wrote This Book

1. The term "root cause(s)," which appears throughout this book, refers to underlying agents of chronic inflammation, e.g., toxic heavy metals, chemicals, environmental toxins, nutritional deficiencies, sedentary lifestyles, sleep issues, hormone imbalances, chronic infections, stress, and others. These are the hidden triggers that can lead to chronic health conditions unless they are identified and treated in their early stages

Introduction

1. Y.H. El-Hayek, R.E. Wiley, C.P. Khoury, R.P. Daya, C. Ballard, A.R. Evans, M. Karran, J.L. Molinuevo, M. Norton, and A. Atri (2019). "Tip of the Iceberg: Assessing the Global Socioeconomic Costs of Alzheimer's Disease and Related Dementias and Strategic Implications for Stakeholders." *Journal of Alzheimer's disease: JAD, 70*(2), 323–341, https://content.iospress.com/articles/journal-of-alzheimers-disease/jad190426.

2. Dan Watts, MD, is board-certified in integrative medicine, by the American Board of Anti-Aging and Regenerative Medicine, the American Board of Clinical Metal Toxicology, and the American Naturopathic Medical Board. For more information on The Renewal Point in Sarasota, Florida, see https://therenewalpoint.com/.

Chapter 3: Seasons of Despair

1. "Hashimoto encephalopathy," National Institutes of Health, Genetic and Rare Diseases, https://rarediseases.info.nih.gov/diseases/8570/hashimoto-encephalopathy.

2. Roger Ebert, *Awakenings,* review of the film starring Robin Williams about patients suffering from neurological afflictions starring Robin Williams, December 20, 1990, https://rogerebert.com/reviews/awakenings-1990. Ironically, years later Williams would be stricken with a mysterious, neurological illness.

Chapter 4: Continuing Concerns

1. UNC School of Medicine. "Neuropsychological Evaluation FAQ—What is neuropsychology?," UNC Department of Neurology, Chapel Hill, NC, https://med.unc.edu/neurology/divisions/movement-disorders/npsycheval/.

Chapter 5: A Toxic Illness Diagnosis

1. Ritchie C. Shoemaker, MD, with James Schaller, MD and Patti Schmidt, *Mold Warriors: Fighting America's Hidden Health Threat* (Tyler, TX: Gateway Press, 2005), 92.

2. Ibid., 93.

3. Ibid., 3.

4. Ritchie C. Shoemaker, MD, *Surviving Mold: Life in the Era of Dangerous Buildings.* (Otter Bay Books; 2010).

5. SurvivingMold.com. "The Biotoxin Pathway," http://survivingmold.com/diagnosis/the-biotoxin-pathway.

6. Neil Nathan, MD, **TOXIC**—*Heal Your Body from Mold Toxicity, Lyme Disease, Multiple Chemical Sensitivities, and Chronic Environmental Illness,* (Las Vegas, NV: Victory Belt Publishing, 2018), 232.

7. Linlin Chen, Huldan Deng, Hengmin Cui, Jing Fang, Zhical Zuo, Junliang Deng, Yinglun Li, Xun Wang, and Ling Zhao, "Inflammatory responses and inflammation-associated diseases in organs," *Oncotarget* 2018; 9: 7204-7218, https://www.oncotarget.com/article/23208/text/.

8. John E. Upledger, (July 2004). "Toxic Brain Injury (Encephalopathy)," *Massage Today,* Volume 04, Issue 07, July 2004, International Alliance of Healthcare Educators, https://www.iahe.com/docs/articles/2852_001.pdf.

9. Ibid.

Chapter 6: Challenges of an Accurate Diagnosis

1. Charles W. Schmidt, "Questions Persist: Environmental Factors in Autoimmune Disease," which quoted Stanley P. Finger, PhD, former chairman of the AARDA (now known as the Autoimmune Association) board of directors, *Environmental Health Perspectives,* 2011, 119(6), A249–A253, https://ehp.niehs.nih.gov/doi/full/10.1289/ehp.119-a248.

2. *TOXIC,* 39.

3. Ritchie C. Shoemaker, *Surviving Mold: Life in the Era of Dangerous Buildings,* (Baltimore, MD: Otter Bay Books, 2010), 53.

4. Ibid. p. 54-55.

5. A.W. Campbell, J.D. Thrasher, M.R. Gray, and A. Zojdani, "Mold and mycotoxins: effects on the neurological and immune systems in humans," *Advances in Applied Microbiology, 55,* 2004, 375–406, https://pubmed.ncbi.nlm.nih.gov/15350803/.

6. W.M. Haschek and K.A. Voss, "Safety assessment including current and emerging issues in toxicologic pathology," *Handbook of Toxicologic Pathology* (Third Edition), (Cambridge, MA: Academic Press, 2013), 1249.

7. Toxic Mold Foundation, "Doctors' diagnosis on mold may complicate the problem," https://toxicmoldfoundation.com/240.html.

8. *Surviving Mold,* 26.

Chapter 7: Transformational Turning Points

1. *Mold Warriors,* xxxvi-xxxvii.

2. Ibid., 80-81.

Chapter 8: The Unraveling of a Beloved Man

1. "Toxins and Infections," Neuro-Luminance Brain Health Centers, https://neuro-luminance.com/conditions/toxins-and-infections/, accessed January 16, 2021.

2. Ibid.

3. A Quantitative Electroencephalograph (QEEG), which maps the areas of the brain exhibiting abnormal activity, can predict what type of symptoms a patient may likely experience as a result. A QEEG can identify brainwaves, their amplitude, location and coherence (quality of communication between regions of the brain), and speed of thinking. These are all crucial patterns involved in optimum mental functioning. The QEEG information can be interpreted and used by experts as a clinical tool to evaluate brain function, and to track the changes in brain function due to various interventions such as neurofeedback or medication.

4. Jonathan T. Stewart, (August 2006). "The frontal/subcortical dementias—Common dementing illnesses associated with prominent and disturbing behavioral changes." *Geriatrics,* August 2006, Volume 61, Number 8, 24-225, https://pubmed.ncbi.nlm.nih.gov/16901194/.

Chapter 10: A Difference of Opinions

1. Jeffrey L. Cummings, MD and D. Frank Benson, MD, "Subcortical dementia: Review of an emerging concept." *Archives of neurology* 1984: 41(8), 874–879, https://jamanetwork.com/journals/jamaneurology/article-abstract/583337.

2. "Frontal/subcortical dementias—Common dementing illnesses associated with prominent and disturbing behavioral changes."

Chapter 11: The Roller Coaster Ride of Cognition and Care

1. "Bell's Palsy Fact Sheet," National Institute of Neurological Disorders and Stroke, https://www.ninds.nih.gov/Disorders/Patient-Caregiver-Education/Fact-Sheets/Bells-Palsy-Fact-Sheet.

2. "Lewy body dementia," Mayo Clinic, https://www.mayoclinic.org/diseases-conditions/lewy-body-dementia/diagnosis-treatment/drc-20352030.

3. Dr. James Ellison, "Is It Alzheimer's Disease or Lewy Body Dementia?" BrightFocus Foundation, https://www.brightfocus.org/alzheimers/article/it-alzheimers-disease-or-lewy-body-dementia, accessed May 11, 2021.

4. Carol A.C. Coupland PhD, Trevor Hill MSc; Tom Dening MD, Richard Morriss MD, Michael Moore MSc; and Julia Hippisley-Cox MD, "Anticholinergic drug exposure and the risk of dementia: A nested case-control study," *JAMA Internal Medicine* 2019;179(8): 1084–1093, https://jamanetwork.com/journals/jamainternalmedicine/fullarticle/2736353.

5. Sujit Rambhade, Anup Chakarborty, Anand Shrivastava, Umesh K. Patil, and Ashish Rambhade, "A survey on polypharmacy and use of inappropriate medications." *Toxicology International*, January 19, 2012, (1)68-73, https://pubmed.ncbi.nlm.nih.gov/22736907/.

6. Ibid.

7. Ibid.

8. Lisa Cooke, "It's Showtime!" Lewy Warriors.wordpress.com (blogpost), February 22, 2016, https://lewywarriors.wordpress.com/2016/02/22/its-showtime/.

Chapter 12: Making Peace from Our Journey

1. Dale E. Bredesen MD, *The End of Alzheimer's—The First Program to Prevent and Reverse Cognitive Decline* (New York: Penguin Publishing Group, 2017), 10.

2. Pharmacologist Joe Graedon and medical anthropologist Terrry Graedon host *The People's Pharmacy* Radio Program on North Carolina Public Radio, which can be found at https://www.npr.org/podcasts/381444414/the-people-s-pharmacy-radio-program. The episode I heard aired on September 10, 2017.

3. *The End of Alzheimer's,* 107.

4. Dale E. Bredesen MD, "Inhalational Alzheimer's disease: an unrecognized—and treatable—epidemic," *Aging,* Volume 8, Issue 2, 304–313, https://www.aging-us.com/article/100896.

5. Ibid.

6. Margaret Christensen MD, transcripts from The Toxic Mold Summit (Dallas, TX: Health Means, 2020), 197. For more information, see https://toxicmold.byhealthmeans.com/.

Chapter 13: Bodies on Fire

1. Mark Hyman MD, *The UltraMind Solution: The Simple Way to Defeat Depression, Overcome Anxiety, and Sharpen Your Mind* (New York: Scribner, 2009), 235.

2. Irvin was quoted in the book, *The Hundred-Year Lie—How Food and Medicine are Destroying Your Health,* by Randall Fitzgerald (New York: Dutton/Penguin Group, 2006), 33.

3. *The UltraMind Solution,* 216.

4. Pizzorno was quoted by Erik Goldman in the article, "Death and toxins: Tackling the main driver of chronic disease" in the May 17, 2017 issue of *Holistic Primary Care,* https://holisticprimarycare.net/topics/environomics/death-and-toxins-tackling-the-main-driver-of-chronic-disease/. He was citing material from Pizzorno's book, *The Toxin Solution: How Hidden Poisons in the Air, Water, Food, and Products We Use Are Destroying Our Health—AND WHAT WE CAN DO TO FIX IT* (New York: HarperCollins Publishers, 2017).

Chapter 14: Root Cause Realities

1. "Body burden—The pollution in newborns," Environmental Working Group, July 14, 2005, ewg.org/research/body-burden-pollution-newborns.

2. Randall Fitzgerald, *The Hundred Year Lie: How to Protect Yourself from the Chemicals that Are Destroying Your Health* (New York: Dutton/Penguin Group, 2006), 21-22.

3. "Death and toxins: Tackling the main driver of chronic disease."

4. Ibid.

5. Ibid.

6. Ibid.

7. *The Toxin Solution: How Hidden Poisons in the Air, Water, Food, and Products We Use Are Destroying Our Health—AND WHAT WE CAN DO TO FIX IT, 23-24.*

8. Paula Baille-Hamilton, *Toxic Overload: A Doctor's Plan for Combating the Illnesses Caused by Chemicals in Our Foods, Our Homes, and Our Medicine Cabinets* (New York: Avery, 2005).

9. "EPA Inventory Update Reporting program," https://www.worldometers.info/view/toxchem/, accessed May 5, 2020.

10. Ibid.

11. Centers for Disease Control and Prevention, *Fourth National Report on Human Exposure to Environmental Chemicals,* tables updated January 2019, https://cfpub.epa.gov/ncea/risk/hhra/recordisplay.cfm, accessed May 20, 2021.

12. "Personal Care Products Safety Act would improve cosmetics safety," Environmental Working Group, October 2019, https://www.ewg.org/Personal-Care-Products-Safety-Act-Would-Improve-Cosmetics-Safety.

13. Scott Faber, "The Top Twenty Toxic Chemicals and Contaminants in Cosmetics," Environmental Working Group, April 3, 2019, https://www./ewg.org/californiacosmetics/toxic20.

14. "EWG's Guide to Sunscreens," Environmental Working Group, https://www.ewg.org/sunscreen/, accessed May 20, 2021.

15. "The Toxic Twenty Cosmetic Ingredients and Contaminants," Environmental Working Group, https://www.ewg.org/sites/default/files/u352/EWG_Toxic20List_C02.pdf?_ga=2.92349721.522007275.1575981095-64794089.1575981095.

16. Britt Erikson, "US FDA finalizes hand sanitizer rule," *Chemical and Engineering News,* April 11, 2019, https://cen.acs.org/safety/consumer-safety/US-FDA-finalizes-hand-sanitizer/97/web/2019/04.

17. Phillipe Grandjean MD, and Philip J. Landrigan MD, "Neurobehavioural effects of developmental toxicity," *The Lancet/Neurology,* March 2014, https://www.thelancet.com/journals/laneur/article/PIIS1474-4422(13)70278-3/fulltext.

18. Donna Jackson Nakazawa, *The Autoimmune Epidemic: Bodies Gone Haywire in a World Out of Balance—and the Cutting-Edge Science that Promises Hope,* (New York: Touchstone Books, 2008), 55.

19. Jesse Hirsch, "Heavy metals in baby food: What you need to know," *Consumer Reports,* August 16, 2018, https://www.consumerreports.org/food-safety/heavy-metals-in-baby-food/.

20. Janet K. Kern, David A. Geier, Geir Bjørklund, Paul G. King, Kristin G. Homme, Boyd E. Haley, Lisa K. Sykes, and Mark R. Geier, "Evidence supporting a link between dental amalgams and chronic illness, fatigue, depression, anxiety, and suicide." *Neuro endocrinology letters,* 35(7), 537–552, 2014, https://pubmed.ncbi.nlm.nih.gov/25617876/.

21. Gerhard Winneke, "Developmental aspects of environmental neurotoxicology: Lessons from lead and polychlorinated biphenyls," *Journal of the Neurological Sciences,* Volume 308, Issues 1-2, September 2011, 9-15, https://www.sciencedirect.com/science/article/abs/pii/S0022510X11002814.

22. Keith Berndtson, MD, "Chronic Inflammatory Response Syndrome, overview, diagnosis, and treatment," 2013, https://www.hoffmancentre.com/wp-content/uploads/pdfs/am/Chronic_Inflammatory_Response_Syndrome.pdf.

23. Aarane M. Ratnaseelan, Irene Tsilioni, and Theoharis C. Theoharides, "Effects of Mycotoxins on Neuropsychiatric Symptoms and Immune Processes," *Clinical Therapeutics,* Volume 40, Number 6, 903-917, June 5, 2018, https://pubmed.ncbi.nlm.nih.gov/29880330/.

24. *The End of Alzheimer's,* 152.

25. Quote by Dr. Tom O'Bryan, interviewed for *The Toxic Mold Summit* docuseries airing August 2020 and appearing in *The Toxic Mold Summit Transcripts,* 96.

26. "The dirty secret of government drinking water standards," Environmental Working Group, from *EWG's Tap Water Database—2019 Update,* October 2019, https://www.ewg.org/tapwater/.

27. Melissa Denchak, "Flint water crisis: Everything you need to know," National Resources Defense Council, November 8, 2018, https://www.nrdc.org/stories/flint-water-crisis-everything-you-need-know.

28. "Water Fluoridation Data and Statistics," Centers for Disease Control, January 13, 2020, https://www.cdc.gov/fluoridation/statistics/index.htm.

29. "NRC's Recommendations," National Research Council (2006), Fluoride Action Network, https://fluoridealert.org/researchers/nrc/recommendations/.

30. "Impact of fluoride on neurological development in children," Harvard School of Public Health, July 25, 2012, https://www.hsph.harvard.edu/news/features/fluoride-childrens-health-grandjean-choi/.

31. Stuart Cooper, "Unprecedented lawsuit could end water fluoridation in U.S. based on neurotoxicity studies," Fluoride Action Network, June 13, 2017, http://fluoridealert.org/news/unprecedented-lawsuit-could-end-water-fluoridation-in-us-based-on-neurotoxicity-studies/.

32. "TSCA Trial," Fluoride Action Network, http://fluoridealert.org/issues/tsca-fluoride-trial/, accessed May 21, 2021.

33. Arjun Walia, "Dr. Martin Pall: Putting in tens of millions of 5G antennae without a single biological test of safety has got to be the stupidest idea anyone has had in the history of the world," *EM Facts Consultancy,* February 24, 2019, https://www.emfacts.com/2019/02/dr-martin-pall-putting-in-tens-of-millions-of-5g-antennae-without-a-single-biological-test-of-safety-has-got-to-be-about-the-stupidest-idea-anyone-has-had-in-the-history-of-the-world/.

34. Zi-cheng Sun, Jian-long Ge, Bin Guo, Jun Guo, et. al., "Extremely Low Frequency Electromagnetic Fields Facilitate Vesicle Endocytosis by Increasing Presynaptic Calcium Channel Expression at a Central Synapse," *Scientific Reports 6,* article number 21774, February 18, 2016, https://www.nature.com/articles/srep21774.

35. "IARC Classifies Radiofrequency Electromagnetic Fields as Possibly Carcinogenic to Humans," World Health Organization, International Agency for Research on Cancer, May 31, 2011, https://www.iarc.who.int/wp-content/uploads/2018/07/pr208_E.pdf.

36. "Cellphone Frequency Radiation Studies," National Toxicology Program, National Institute of Environmental Sciences, August 2020, https://www.niehs.nih.gov/health/materials/cell_phone_radiofrequency_radiation_studies_508.pdf.

37. Erina Cirino, "Should you be worried about EMF exposure?" *Healthline.com,* March 8, 2019, https://www.healthline.com/health/emf#TOC_TITLE_HDR_1.

38. Theresa Dale, PhD, CCN, "Heavy metal toxicity increases your risk of electromagnetic sensitivity," *Doctor's Corner*, September 11, 2012, https://www.wellnesscenter.net/ heavy-metal-toxicity-increases-your-risk-of-electromagnetic-sensitivity/.

39. "Veteran MD Drops Bombshell About 5G Technology Dangers at 5G Hearing," YouTube, October 4, 2018, Sharon Goldberg testifying in opposition to Michigan Senate Bills 637 and 894 pertaining to small cell towers legislation, https://www.youtube.com/watch?v=1Qt5B39LB7c.

40. "Death and toxins: Tackling the main driver of chronic disease."

41. *The End of Alzheimer's,* 197.

42. Cleveland Clinic, "What happens when your immune system gets stressed out?" March 1, 2017, https://health.clevelandclinic.org/ what-happens-when-your-immune-system-gets-stressed-out/.

43. Ying Chen and John Lyga, "Brain-skin connection: stress, inflammation and skin aging," *Inflammation & Allergy Drug Targets* 2014, 13(3), 177–190, https:// pubmed.ncbi.nlm.nih.gov/24853682/.

44. Ocean Robbins, "12 detoxifying foods to help your body heal," January 11, 2019, Food Revolution Network, https://foodrevolution.org/blog/ detoxifying-foods/.

45. *The Hundred Year Lie,* 98.

46. Quoted on *Eat4Earth* online video documentary, "Heal your body, Heal the planet," https://www.eat4earth.org/upgrade-physical-digital-event/.

47. Donald R. Davis, Melvin D. Epp, and Hugh D. Riordan, "Changes in USDA food composition data for 43 garden crops, 1950 to 1999," *Journal of the American College of Nutrition,* December 23, 2004, (6):66982, 669-682, https://pubmed. ncbi.nlm.nih.gov/15637215/.

48. EWG Science Team, Environmental Working Group, "*EWG's 2021 Shopper's Guide for Pesticides in Produce*™," March 17, 2021, https://www.ewg.org/ foodnews/summary.php.

49. Ibid.

50. Alexis Temkin, PhD and toxicologist, "More than half of kale samples tainted by possible cancer-causing pesticide," Environmental Working Group, March 20, 2019, https://www.ewg.org/foodnews/kale.php.

51. "About Genetically-Engineered Foods," Center for Food Safety, https://www. centerforfoodsafety.org/issues/311/ge-foods/about-ge-foods, accessed May 24, 2021.

52. Ibid., "Overview—Primary food crops," *GMO Awareness.com.*

53. Ibid., "U.S. polls on GE food labeling."

54. "BE disclosure," Agricultural Marketing Service, USDA, https://www.ams.usda.gov/rules-regulations/be, accessed May 24, 2021.

55. "New 'bioengineered' labeling rule will cause further confusion," *National Sustainable Agriculture Coalition Blog,* January 8, 2019, https://sustainableagriculture.net/blog/bioengineered-labeling-rule-will-cause-further-confusion/.

56. "10 reasons to avoid GM foods," *Health Science Research,* February 18, 2018, https://www.health-science.com/gmo/.

57. Swanson, N.L., Leu, A., Abrahamson, J., & Wallet, B. (2014, November). "Genetically engineered crops, glyphosate and the deterioration of health in the United States of America." *Journal of Organic Systems* 2014, 9(2), https://jeffreydachmd.com/wp-content/uploads/2015/04/Genetically-engineered-crops-glyphosate-deterioration-health-United-States-Swanson-J-Organic-Systems-2014.pdf.

58. Ibid.

59. Anthony Samsel and Stephanie Seneff, "Glyphosate's suppression of cytochrome P450 enzymes and amino acid biosynthesis by the gut microbiome: Pathways to modern diseases," *Entropy,* Volume 15, Issue 4, 2013, 1416-1463, https://www.mdpi.com/1099-4300/15/4/1416.

60. David Perlmutter MD, *Grain Brain: The Surprising Truth about Wheat, Carbs, and Sugar - - Your Brain's Silent Killers* (New York: Little, Brown and Company), 8.

61. *Grain Brain,* 52-53, quote from Marios Hadjivassiliou referencing research in *The Lancet.*

62. Stacy Malkan, "Aspartame: Decades of Science Point to Serious Health Risks," US RTK U.S. Right to Know, November 15, 2020, https://usrtk.org/sweeteners/aspartame_health_risks/.

63. Arbind Kumar Choudhary and Yeong Yeh Lee, "Neurophysiological symptoms and aspartame: What is the connection?" *Nutritional Neuroscience,* Volume 21, 2018, (5), 306–316, https://www.tandfonline.com/doi/abs/10.1080/1028415X.2017.1288340?journalCode=ynns20.

64. "Aspartame," National Center for Biotechnology Information, *PubChem Compound* Summary for CID 134601, https://pubchem.ncbi.nlm.nih.gov/compound/Aspartame, accessed June 4, 2021.

65. Matthew P. Pase PhD, Jayndra J. Himali PhD, Alexa S. Beiser PhD, Hugo J. Aparicio MD, Claudia L. Satizabal PhD, and MD Paul F. Jacques DSc, "Sugar and artificially sweetened beverages and the risks of incident stroke and dementia,"

Stroke, Issue 48: 1139–1146, April 20, 2017, https://www.ahajournals.org/doi/full/10.1161/STROKEAHA.116.016027.

66. Ian A. Myles "Fast food fever: reviewing the impacts of the Western diet on immunity," *Nutrition Journal,* 13, Article number: 61 (2014), June 17, 2014, https://nutritionj.biomedcentral.com/articles/10.1186/1475-2891-13-61.

67. Kyla Dunn, "Fooling with Nature: How do hormones work?" *Frontline,* 2014, https://www.pbs.org/wgbh/pages/frontline/shows/nature/etc/hormones.html.

68. *Grain Brain,* 132.

69. Jeffrey A. Woods, Kenneth R. Wilund, Stephen A. Martin, and Brandon M. Kistler, "Exercise, inflammation and aging," *Aging and Disease,* February 3, 2012, (1): 130–140, https://www.ncbi.nlm.nih.gov/pmc/articles/PMC3320801/.

70. Rachel Rettner, "How Exercise Fights Inflammation," *LiveScience,* July 31, 2017, https://www.livescience.com/59988-exercise-fights-inflammation.html.

71. A. E. Autry and L. M. Monteggia LM. "Brain-derived neurotrophic factor and neuropsychiatric disorders." *Pharmacol Rev.* 2012;64(2):238-258. doi:10.1124/pr.111.005108.

72. "Brain basics: Understanding sleep," National Institute of Neurological Disorders and Stroke, https://www.ninds.nih.gov/Disorders/patient-caregiver-education/Understanding-sleep, accessed May 24, 2021.

73. Anne Tergesen, "What Science Tells Us About Preventing Dementia," *Wall Street Journal: Journal Reports: Retirement,* November 18, 2019, https://www.wsj.com/articles/what-science-tells-us-about-preventing-dementia-11574004600.

74. Dale E. Bredesen, MD, *The End of Alzheimer's Program—The First Protocol to Enhance Cognition and Reverse Decline at Any Age,* (Avery, New York, 2020), 295.

75. William L. Stone, Hajira Basit, and Bracken Burns, *Pathology, Inflammation,* Online: StatsPearl Publishing, last updated December 4, 2020, https://www.ncbi.nlm.nih.gov/books/NBK534820/.

Chapter 15: The Rise of Autoimmune Issues

1. Autoimmune Association, https://www.aarda.org/who-we-are/our-mission/, accessed May 24, 2021.

2. Stephanie Watson, "Autoimmune Diseases: Types, Symptoms, Causes, and More: What is an autoimmune disease?" *Healthline,* updated March 26, 2019, https://www.healthline.com/health/autoimmune-disorders.

3. Colleen Travers , "Why Autoimmune Diseases Are on the Rise," (quote attributed to George Rutledge, MD, PhD), *Shape,* December 13, 2016, https://www.shape.com/lifestyle/mind-and-body/why-autoimmune-diseases-are-rise.

4. Ibid.

5. "There are more than 100 Autoimmune Diseases," Autoimmune Association, https://www.aarda.org/diseaselist/, accessed May 24, 2021.

6. Charles W. Schmidt, "Questions Persist: Environmental Factors in Autoimmune Disease," *Environmental Health Perspectives,* June 2011, 119(6): A248-A253, https://www.ncbi.nlm.nih.gov/pmc/articles/PMC3114837/.

7. Noel R. Rose, MD, PhD, "The Common Thread: How Autoimmune Diseases Are Related," Autoimmune Association, https://www.aarda.org/wp-content/uploads/2019/12/Common-Thread-Brochure.pdf.

8. *The Autoimmune Epidemic,* 72.

9. Jean Robbins, "Healing: The Body is the Last to Know—Part 1, www.autoimmunityjr.org, August 26, 2015, https://autoimmunityjr.org/healing-the-body-is-the-last-to-know-part-i/ accessed October 15, 2021.

10. Erin Magner, "The on-the-rise autoimmune diseases that every woman needs to know about." *Well + Good.com.* September 14, 2016, https://www.wellandgood.com/autoimmune-diseases-treat-naturally-women/.

11. "ACE Overview and Mission," Autoimmunity Centers of Excellence, last updated January 27, 2020, https://www.autoimmunitycenters.org/mission.php.

12. "The Common Thread: How Autoimmune Diseases Are Related."

13. Rosemarie G. Ramos and Kenneth Olden, "Gene-Environment Interactions in the Development of Complex Disease Phenotypes, *International Journal of Environmental Research and Public Health 2008,* 5(1), 4–11, https://www.mdpi.com/1660-4601/5/1/4.

14. *Mold Warriors,* 96.

15. "The role of the gut microbiome," media briefing, *SciLine,* August 21, 2019, https://www.sciline.org/health-medicine/gut-microbiome/.

16. Arianana K. DeGruttola BS, Daren Low PhD, Atsushi Mizoguchi MD/PhD, and Emiko Mizoguchi, "Current understanding of dysbiosis in disease in human and animal models." *Inflammatory Bowel Diseases,* Volume 22, Issue 5: 1137-1150, May 1, 2016, https://academic.oup.com/ibdjournal/article/22/5/1137/4561797.

17. R.B. Ashman and J.M. Papadimitrou, "Production and function of cytokines in natural and acquired immunity to Candida albicans infection," *Microbiology Reviews,* December 1995; 59(4): 646–672, https://www.ncbi.nlm.nih.gov/pmc/articles/PMC239393/.

18. Stephen S. Dominy, Casey Lynch, et. al., "*Porphyromonas gingivalis* in Alzheimer's disease brains: Evidence for disease causation and treatment with small-molecule inhibitors," *Science Advances,* Volume 5, No. 1, January 23, 2019, https://advances.sciencemag.org/content/5/1/eaau3333.

19. Sara Adaes, PhD, "How the gut microbiota influences our immune system." *Neurohacker Collective,* July 8, 2019, https://neurohacker.com/how-the-gut-microbiota-influences-our-immune-system.

20. Marcelo Campos, MD "Leaky gut: What is it, and what does it mean for you?" *Harvard Health Blog,* September 22, 2017, https://www.health.harvard.edu/blog/leaky-gut-what-is-it-and-what-does-it-mean-for-you-2017092212451.

21. Ibid.

22. Kristiana Xhima, Danielle Weber-Adrian, and Joseph Silburt, "Glutamate Induces Blood–Brain Barrier Permeability through Activation of N-Methyl-D-Aspartate Receptors," *Journal of Neuroscience,* December 7, 2016, 36 (49) pp. 12296-12298, https://www.jneurosci.org/content/36/49/12296.

23. Ibid.

24. The Institute for Functional Medicine, "Rise of autoimmune disease linked to intestinal permeability," https://www.ifm.org/news-insights/ai-rise-autoimmune-disease-linked-intestinal-permeability/, accessed May 25, 2021.

25. Ellen Barlow, "Celiac Disease and the Unforeseen Path to Discovery," Massachusetts General Hospital, 2014, https://giving.massgeneral.org/celiac-disease-unforeseen-path-discovery/.

26. Heather B. Patisaul and Wendy Jefferson, "The pros and cons of phytoestrogens," *Frontiers in Neuroendocrinology,* Volume 31, Issue 4, October 2010, 400-419, https://www.sciencedirect.com/science/article/abs/pii/S0091302210000257.

27. Isabell Wentz with Marta Nowosadzka, *Hashimoto's Thyroiditis—Lifestyle Interventions for Finding and Treating the Root Cause* (Des Plaines, IL: Wentz LLC), 144.

28. Ibid., 129.

29. Ibid., 42-43.

Chapter 16: Gut Issues: Ground Zero for Inflammation

1. Emeran Mayer, MD, *The Mind-Gut Connection—How the Hidden Conversation Within Our Bodies Impacts Our Mood, Our Choices, and Our Overall Health* (New York: Harper Wave, 2016), 95-96.

2. Ibid., 250.

3. Adam Hadhazy, "Think Twice: How the Gut's 'Second Brain' Influences Mood and Well-Being," *Scientific-American,* February 12, 2010, https://www.scientificamerican.com/article/gut-second-brain/.

4. Dr. Siri Carpenter, "That Gut Feeling," American Psychological Association, September 2012, Volume 43, No. 8, https://www.apa.org/monitor/2012/09/gut-feeling.

5. Michael C. Toh and Emma Allen-Vercoe, "The human gut microbiota with reference to autism spectrum disorder: considering the whole as more than a sum of its parts," *Microbial Ecology in Health and Disease*, 2015, 26: 10.3402/mehd.v26.26309, https://www.ncbi.nlm.nih.gov/pmc/articles/PMC4310852/.

6. Dale E. Bredesen, MD, *The End of Alzheimer's Program*, 291.

Chapter 17: Neurotoxicity—Toxic Assault of the Brain

1. Dr. Raymond Singer and Dana Darby Johnson, "Recognizing Neurotoxicity." *Trial,* Vol. 42, Number 3, 62, February 28, 2006, copyright: The Association of Trial Lawyers of America, reprinted with permission. For more information on Dr. Singer, http://neurotox.com/.

2. John Neustadt and Steve R. Pieczenik, "Medication-induced mitochondrial damage and disease,*" Molecular Nutrition & Food Research,* Volume 52, Issue 7, 780-788, July 14, 2008, https://onlinelibrary.wiley.com/doi/abs/10.1002/mnfr.200700075.

3. Abigail Shrier, "Standing against psychiatry's crazes," *Wall Street Journal, WSJ/Opinion,* May 3, 2019, https://www.wsj.com/articles/standing-against-psychiatrys-crazes-11556920766.

4. "Recognizing Neurotoxicity."

5. Peter Bengsten and Danwatch, (October 26, 2012), "Toxic chemicals used for leather production poisoning India's tannery's workers," *The Ecologist,* October 26, 2012, https://theecologist.org/2012/oct/26/toxic-chemicals-used-leather-production-poisoning-indias-tannery-workers.

6. "Metals Urine Test," The Great Plains Laboratory, Inc., Lenaxa, KS, https://www.greatplainslaboratory.com/metals-urine-test, accessed May 26, 2021.

7. "Toxins and Infections," Neuro-Luminance Brain Health Centers, neuro-luminance.com/conditions/toxins-and-infections/, accessed July 20, 2020.

8. Keith Berndtson, MD, "Chronic Inflammatory Response Syndrome—Overview, Diagnosis and Treatment," 2013, https://hoffmancentre.com/wp-content/ uploads/pdfs/am/Chronic_Inflammatory_Response_Syndrome.pdf, accessed March 15, 2019.

9. "Lead poisoning: Diagnosis and Treatment," Mayo Clinic, https://www.mayoclinic.org/diseases-conditions/lead-poisoning/diagnosis-treatment/drc-20354723, accessed May 26, 2021.

10. Joseph Pizzorno, "Is Challenge Testing Valid for Assessing Body Metal Burden?" *Integrative Medicine,* Volume 14, No. 4, 8-14, August 2014, https://www.ncbi.nlm.nih.gov/pmc/articles/PMC4712860/.

11. Sherry A. Rogers, MD, *Detoxify or Die* (San Francisco: Prestige Publications, 2002).

12. S. Porru and L. Alessio, (1996, February 1). "The Use of Chelating Agents in Occupational Lead Poisoning." *Occupational Medicine,* Volume 46, Issue 1, 41–48, February 1, 1996, https://academic.oup.com/occmed/article/46/1/41/1410785.

13. "Fact Sheet on Mercury," Agency for Toxic Substances and Disease Registry, IOAMT, https://iaomt.org/wp-content/uploads/Unit-2-BDHA-REQUIRED.pdf, updated October 10, 2019.

14. *"Porphyromonas gingivalis* in Alzheimer's disease brains."

15. Neil Nathan, MD, *Toxic: Heal Your Body from Mold Toxicity, Lyme Disease, Multiple Chemical Sensitivities, and Chronic Environmental Illness* (Las Vegas, NV: Victory Belt Publishing, 2018), 187.

16. "Dental Amalgam Mercury Fillings and Dangers to Human Health," International Academy of Oral Medicine & Toxicology, https://iaomt.org/resources/dental-mercury-facts/amalgam-fillings-danger-human-health/?cn-reloaded=1, accessed May 26, 2021.

17. "The Safe Mercury Amalgam Removal Technique (SMART), International Academy of Oral Medicine & Toxicology, https://iaomt.org/resources/safe-removal-amalgam-fillings/, accessed May 26, 2021.

18. "Oral Health Integration and Biological Dentistry," IAOMT.org, https://iaomt.org/about-iaomt/oral-health-integration/, accessed October 12, 2021.

Chapter 18: Conventional Medicine vs. Functional/Integrative Medicine

1. "The Functional Medicine Approach," Institute of Functional Medicine, https://www.ifm.org/functional-medicine/what-is-functional-medicine/, accessed May 27, 2021.

2. Dr. Anita Sadaty, "Functional Medicine vs. Conventional Medicine," https://www.drsadaty.com/, accessed May 27, 2021.

3. "Introduction," *Academic Consortium of Academic Health Centers for Integrative Medicine,* https://imconsortium.org/about/introduction/, accessed April 8, 2021.

4. "The Functional Medicine Approach."

Chapter 19: Revelations from a Functional Perspective

1. "The No-Amylose Diet," *Journey Toward Health,* http://www. journeytowardhealth.com/no-amylose-diet/, accessed May 27, 2021.

2. The End of Alzheimer's, 117-118; and "Cognoscopy," Apollo Health https:// apollohealthco.com/cognoscopy/.

3. Ann Wigmore developed the Living Foods Lifestyle˚ to overcome disease and improve the quality of life. Quote from https://www.goodreads.com/author/ quotes/385454.Ann_Wigmore, accessed May 27, 2021.

4. *The Toxin Solution,* 36.

5. Esther Crain, "21 Important Facts about Vitamin B$_{12}$ Deficiency," *Health.com,* updated December 20, 2019, https://www.health.com/ nutrition/21-important-facts-about-vitamin-b12-deficiency.

6. Kathleen Mikkelsen, Lily Stojanovska, and Vasso Apostolopoulos, "The Effects of Vitamin B in Depression," *Current Medicinal Chemistry,* 2016: 23: 4317, doi. org/10.2174/0929867323666160920110810, https://pubmed.ncbi.nlm.nih. gov/27655070/.

7. Bradley A. Maron MD, and Joseph Loscalzo MD, "The Treatment of Hyperhomocysteinemia," *Annual Review of Medicine,* 2009: 60: 39–54, https://www.ncbi.nlm.nih.gov/pmc/articles/PMC2716415/.

8. Gwenaelle Douaud, Helga Refsum, Celeste de Jager, Robin Jacoby, Thomas E. Nichols, Stephen M. Smith, and A. David Smith, "Preventing Alzheimer's disease-related gray matter atrophy by B-vitamin treatment." *Proceedings of the National Academy of Sciences of the United States of America* June 4, 2013, 110 (23), 9523–9528, https://www.pnas.org/content/110/23/9523.

9. "B Vitamins May Protect Against Damaging Effects of Air Pollution, and Improve Cognition and Psychiatric Health," *Mercola.com,* March 27, 2017, https://articles.mercola.com/sites/articles/archive/2017/03/27/b-vitamins-may-help-protect-against-air-pollution.aspx.

10. Michelle Corey, "Five Strategies to Improve Methylation and Heal from Chronic Illness," *MichelleCorey.com,* August 1, 2015, https://michellecorey.com/ mind-body/methylation-and-glutathione/.

11. *The UltraMind Solution,* 125.

12. Fatma Zehra Kadayifci, Shasha Zheng, and Xuan-Xiagn Pan, "Molecular mechanisms underlying the link between diet and DNA methylation," *International Journal of Molecular Sciences 2018,* 19(12): 4055, https://www.mdpi.com/1422-0067/19/12/4055.

13. Michelle Corey, "Methylation: Why It Matters For Your Immunity, Inflammation & More," *MBG Food, MindBodyGreen.com,* April 9, 2015, https://www.mindbodygreen.com/0-18245/methylation-why-it-matters-for-your-immunity-inflammation-more.html.

14. Donielle Wilson, "How adrenal distress affects MTHFR and methylation," September 14, 2017, *DoctorDoni.com,* https://doctordoni.com/2017/09/how-adrenal-distress-affects-mthfr-and-methylation/.

15. Suzy Cohen, "Methylation problems lead to 100s of diseases," *SuzyCohen.com,* March 26, 2020. suzycohen.com/articles/methylation-problems/. Notation by Suzy Cohen: *A methylation defect does not cause Lyme, a tick-borne biotoxin illness. However, methylation defects reduce the ability to properly detoxify, fight the infection and co-infections, and the damage caused from it."

16. "Basic information about the MTHFR gene," The Permanente Medical Group, 2015, https://mydoctor.kaiserpermanente.org/ncal/Images/GEN_MTHFR_tcm63-938252.pdf.

17. Suzy Cohen, "Methylation Problems Lead to 100s of Diseases." *SuzyCohen.com.* suzycohen.com/articles/methylation-problems/, accessed May 3, 2020.

18. Bruce Lourie and Rick Smith, *Toxin Toxout—Getting Harmful Chemicals Out of Our Bodies and Our World* (New York: St. Martin's Press, 2013), 137.

19. Mehrdad Alirezaei, Christopher C. Kemball, Claudia T. Flynn, Malcom R. Wood, J. Lindsay Whitton, and William B. Kiosses, "Short-term fasting induces profound neuronal autophagy," *Autophagy,* Volume 6, 2010, 702-710, https://www.tandfonline.com/doi/full/10.4161/auto.6.6.12376.

20. *Toxic—Heal Your Body from Mold Toxicity, Lyme Disease, Multiple Chemical Sensitivities, and Chronic Environmental Illness, 231.*

21. Ibid., 229.

22. Kerri-Ann Jennings, "9 Impressive Health Benefits of Chlorella," *Healthline.com,* April 8, 2017, https://www.healthline.com/nutrition/benefits-of-chlorella.

23. Peter Greenlaw, Nicholas Messina, and Drew Greenlaw, *TDOS Syndrome and Solutions (Toxins/Nutritional Deficiencies/ Overweight/Stress),* Austin, TX: Greenlaw Group, 2015), 192.

24. *Surviving Mold,* 24-25.

25. Scott Rollins, MD, is board certified with the American Board of Family Practice and the American Board of Anti-Aging and Regenerative Medicine.

Chapter 20: Smart Choices in Today's Toxic Times

1. *Toxic—Heal Your Body from Mold Toxicity, Lyme Disease, Multiple Chemical Sensitivities, and Chronic Environmental Illness,* 306.

2. "2021 Alzheimer's Disease Facts and Figures," Alzheimer's Association, https://www.alz.org/media/documents/alzheimers-facts-and-figures.pdf, accessed May 28, 2021.

3. "12 detoxifying foods to help your body heal naturally."

4. Ibid.

5. Matthew C.L. Phillips, "Fasting as a therapy in neurological disease," *Nutrients 2019;* 11(10), 2501: published online October 17, 2019, https://www.mdpi.com/2072-6643/11/10/2501.

6. Rafael de Cabo PhD and Mark P. Mattson PhD, "Effects of intermittent fasting on health, aging, and disease," *New England Journal of Medicine,* 381: 2541-2551, December 26, 2019, https://www.nejm.org/doi/full/10.1056/nejmra1905136.

7. Kris Gunnars, "Intermittent Fasting 101—The Ultimate Beginner's Guide," *Healthline.com,* April 20, 2020, https://www.healthline.com/nutrition/intermittent-fasting-guide.

8. Stephen J. Genuis, Detlef Birkholz, Ilia Rodushkin, and Sanjay Beeson, "Blood, Urine, and Sweat (BUS) Study: Monitoring and Elimination of Bioaccumulated Toxic Elements," *Archives of Environmental Contamination and Toxicology* 61, 344–357 (2011), November 6, 2010, https://link.springer.com/article/10.1007/s00244-010-9611-5.

9. "Detox with a Sunlighten Infrared Sauna," *sunlighten.com,* https://www.sunlighten.com/blog/detox-sunlighten-infrared-sauna/, accessed June 1, 2021.

10. Michael R. Hamblin, "Photobiomodulation or low-level laser therapy," *Journal of Biophotonics,* Volume 9, Issue 11-12, 1122–1124, December 14, 2016, https://onlinelibrary.wiley.com/doi/10.1002/jbio.201670113.

11. Janett Hope, "A Review of the Mechanism of Injury and Treatment Approaches for Illness Resulting From Exposure to Water-Damaged Buildings, Mold, and Mycotoxins," *The Scientific World Journal,* Volume 2013, Article ID 767482, April 18, 2013, https://www.hindawi.com/journals/tswj/2013/767482/.

12. Tina Wilson, "Are you detoxing with the correct binders?" *SophiaNutrition.com,* August 6, 2020, https://www.sophianutrition.com/blogs/sophia-life-blog/are-you-detoxing-with-the-correct-binders.

13. Sandra Kraljević Pavelić, Jasmina Simović Medica, Darko Gumbarević, Ana Filosevic, Natasa Pržulj, and Krsimir Pavelić, "Critical Review on Zeolite Clinoptilolite Safety and Medical Applications in vivo," *Frontiers in Pharmacology,* Volume 9: 1350, November 27, 2018, https://www.frontiersin.org/articles/10.3389/fphar.2018.01350/full.

14. "What Do We Know About Diet and Prevention of Alzheimer's Disease?" National Institute on Aging, accessed July 3, 2021, https://www.nia.nih.gov/health/what-do-we-know-about-diet-and-prevention-alzheimers-disease.

15. John F. Cryan and Timothy G. Dinan, "Mind-altering microorganisms: the impact of the gut microbiota on brain and behaviour," *Nature Reviews Neuroscience* 13, 701–712, September 12, 2012, https://www.nature.com/articles/nrn3346.

16. Dr. David Jockers, "6 Ways a Keto Diet Improves Brain Function," DrJockers.com, https://drjockers.com/ketogenic-diet-improves-brain-function/ accessed on October 8, 2021.

17. Joseph Mercola, MD., *Fat for Fuel*, Hay House, Inc., 2017, 36.

18. Dr. David Jockers, "6 Ways A Ketogenic Diet Improves Brain Function," Drjockers.com.

19. Ibid.

20. M. Rusek, R. Pluta, M. Ułamek-Kozioł, & S.J. Czuczwar, "Ketogenic Diet in Alzheimer's Disease." *International Journal of Molecular Sciences*, 20(16), 3892, 2019. https://doi.org/10.3390/ijms20163892Ketogenic Diet in Alzheimer's.

21. Dale E. Bredesen, MD, *The End of Alzheimer's Program—The First Protocol to Enhance Cognition and Reverse Decline at Any Age*, (Avery, New York, 2020, 63-76).

22. "What Do We Know About Diet and Prevention of Alzheimer's Disease?"

23. Ibid.

24. "Foods that Fight Inflammation," *Harvard Health Publishing,* August 29, 2020, https://www.health.harvard.edu/staying-healthy/foods-that-fight-inflammation.

25. Jessie Szalay, "What Are flavonoids?" *LiveScience.com*, October 20, 2015, https://www.livescience.com/52524-flavonoids.html.

26. "Fill up on phytochemicals," *Harvard Health Publishing,* February 2019, https://www.health.harvard.edu/staying-healthy/fill-up-on-phytochemicals.

27. "How Emotions Affect Digestive Health & Why Mindful Eating Can Help Improve Gut Issues," Self-Care for Moms, updated April 30, 2020, https://motherhoodcommunity.com/how-emotions-affect-digestive-health-why-mindful-eating-can-help-improve-gut-issues/.

28. Emilio Ros, "Nuts and novel biomarkers of cardiovascular disease," *The American Journal of Clinical Nutrition,* Volume 89, Issue 5, 1649S-1656S, March 25, 2009, https://academic.oup.com/ajcn/article/89/5/1649S/4596956.

29. Christine Yu, "10 Ways to Reduce Inflammation," *Eating Well,* updated December 17, 2019, https://www.eatingwell.com/article/80991/10-ways-to-reduce-inflammation/.

30. Franziska Spritzler, "The 13 Most Anti-inflammatory Foods You Can Eat," *Healthline.com,* December 19, 2019, https://www.healthline.com/nutrition/13-anti-inflammatory-foods.

31. Daisy Coyle, "Sulforaphane: Benefits, Side Effects, and Food Sources," *Healthline.com,* February 26, 2019, https://www.healthline.com/nutrition/sulforaphane.

32. Lisa Lucas, Aaron Russell, and Russell Keast, "Molecular mechanisms of inflammation. Anti-inflammatory benefits of virgin olive oil and the phenolic compound oleocanthal." *Current Pharmaceutical Design,* 17(8): 754–768, January 1, 2011, https://europepmc.org/article/med/21443487.

33. Jeremy P.E. Spencer, "Flavonoids: modulators of brain function?" *British Journal of Nutrition* (2008), Volume 99, Issue E-Supplement 1, ES60-ES77, https://www.cambridge.org/core/services/aop-cambridge-core/content/view/9AB7C1E220A094F510D8D6A84FD4DC44/S0007114508965776a.pdf/flavonoids-modulators-of-brain-function.pdf.

34. Merel Hazewindus, Guido R. M. M. Haenen, Antje R. Weseler, Aalt Bast, "The anti-inflammatory effect of lycopene complements the antioxidant action of ascorbic acid and α-tocopherol," *Food Chemistry,* May 2012, Volume 132, Issue 2, 954-958, https://doi.org/10.1016/j.foodchem.2011.11.075.

35. Kris Gunnars, BSc, "10 Evidence-Based Benefits of Green Tea," *Healthline.com,* updated April 6, 2020, https://www.healthline.com/nutrition/top-10-evidence-based-health-benefits-of-green-tea.

36. Suzhen Dong, Qingwen Zeng, E. Slobhan Mitchell, Jin Xiu, Yale Duan, Jyoti K. Tiwari, Yinghe Hu, Xiaohua Cao, and Zheng Zhao, "Curcumin Enhances Neurogenesis and Cognition in Aged Rats: Implications for Transcriptional Interactions Related to Growth and Synaptic Plasticity," *PLOS One,* February 16, 2012, https://journals.plos.org/plosone/article?id=10.1371/journal.pone.0031211.

37. Papsupuleti Visweswara Rao and Siew Hua Gan, "Cinnamon: a multifaceted medicinal plant," *Evidence-based complementary and alternative medicine: eCAM,* April 10, 2014, https://pubmed.ncbi.nlm.nih.gov/24817901/.

38. Rohini Terry PhD, Paul Posadzki PhD, Leala K. Watson BSc (Hons), and Edzard Ernst PhD, "The Use of Ginger (Zingiber officinale) for the Treatment of Pain: A Systematic Review of Clinical Trials," *Pain Medicine,* Volume 12, Issue 12, 1808–1818, December 14, 2011, https://academic.oup.com/painmedicine/article/12/12/1808/1846834.

39. "2020 CRN Survey Reveals Focus on Vitamins and Minerals," *Council for Responsible Nutrition,* September 29, 2020, https://www.crnusa.org/newsroom/2020-crn-survey-reveals-focus-vitamins-and-minerals-available-purchase-consumer-survey.

40. "Probiotics may help boost mood and cognitive function," *Harvard Health Publishing,* June 2019, https://www.health.harvard.edu/mind-and-mood/probiotics-may-help-boost-mood-and-cognitive-function.

41. Olivia G. Swann, Michelle Kilpatrick, Monique Breslin, and Wendy H. Oddy, "Dietary fiber and its associations with depression and inflammation." *Nutrition Reviews,* Volume 78, Issue 5, 394–41, May 2020, https://pubmed.ncbi.nlm.nih.gov/31750916/; doi.10.1093/nutrit/nuz072.

42. Arlene Semeco, MS, RD; and Amy Richter, RD, "The 19 best prebiotic foods you should eat," Healthline.com, June 8, 2016 (updated May 11, 2021), https://www.healthline.com/nutrition/19-best-prebiotic-foods.

43. Original story by University College London, "Long-term collateral damage from antibiotics modeled," *Technology Networks,* March 29, 2019, https://www.technologynetworks.com/biopharma/news/how-antibiotics-change-human-microbiome-diversity-long-term-317454.

44. Barbara Jacquelyn Sahakian, Christelle Langley, and Muzaffer Kaser, M. (March 11, 2020). "How chronic stress changes the brain – and what you can do to reverse the damage," *The Conversation,* March 11, 2020, http://theconversation.com/how-chronic-stress-changes-the-brain-and-what-you-can-do-to-reverse-the-damage-133194.

45. Ibid.

46. Mayo Clinic Staff, "Meditation: A simple, fast way to reduce stress," Mayo Clinic, mayoclinic.org/tests-procedures/meditation/indepth/meditation/art-20045858, accessed June 1, 2021.

47. "What Science Tells Us About Preventing Dementia."

48. Ana Sandoiu, "Just 20 minutes of exercise enough to reduce inflammation, study finds," *Medical News Today,* January 16, 2017, https://www.medicalnewstoday.com/articles/315255.

49. "American Heart Association Recommendations for Physical Activity in Adults and Kids," *Heart.org,* April 18, 2018, https://www.heart.org/en/healthy-living/fitness/fitness-basics/aha-recs-for-physical-activity-in-adults.

50. Edward B. Lee, "Obesity, leptin, and Alzheimer's disease." *Annals of the New York Academy of Sciences,* Volume 1243, Issue 1, 15–29, December 2011, https://nyaspubs.onlinelibrary.wiley.com/doi/full/10.1111/j.1749-6632.2011.06274.x.

51. Angela S. Lillehei and Linda L. Halcon, "A systematic review of the effect of inhaled essential oils on sleep," *Journal of Alternative and Complementary Medicine,* Volume 20, Issue 6, 441–451, June 2014, https://pubmed.ncbi.nlm.nih.gov/24720812/.

52. Dr. Michael Breus, "7 Essential Oils for Relaxation and Better Sleep," *The Sleep Doctor,* June 12, 2018, https://thesleepdoctor.com/2018/06/12/7-essential-oils-for-relaxation-and-better-sleep/.

53. "Brain basics: Understanding Sleep," National Institute of Neurological Disorders and Stroke, August 13, 2019, https://www.ninds.nih.gov/Disorders/Patient-Caregiver-Education/Understanding-Sleep.

54. Dr. Emma Seppala, "Connectedness and Health: The Science of Social Connection," Stanford University, The Center for Compassion and Altruism Research and Education, May 8, 2014, http://ccare.stanford.edu/uncategorized/connectedness-health-the-science-of-social-connection-infographic/.

55. "Mold Allergy: What Is a Mold Allergy?" Asthma and Allergy Foundation of America, https://www.aafa.org/mold-allergy/, accessed June 2, 2021.

56. "What is an Air Purifier HEPA Filter?" *AirPurifierRatings.org,* https://air-purifier-ratings.org/learn/hepa-efficiency/, accessed June 2, 2021.

57. "Damp Indoor Spaces and Health (2004)," *The National Academies Press,* The National Academies of Sciences, Engineering, Medicine, https://www.nap.edu/catalog/11011/damp-indoor-spaces-and-health.

58. "Is plastic a threat to your health?" *Harvard Health Publishing,* December 1, 2019, https://www.health.harvard.edu/staying-healthy/is-plastic-a-threat-to-your-health.

59. Daisy Coyle, APD, "Is Nonstick Cookware Like Teflon Safe to Use?" *Healthline.com,* July 13, 2017, https://www.healthline.com/nutrition/nonstick-cookware-safety.

60. "Scientists warn of potential serious health effects of 5G," statement signed by more than 180 scientists from 35 countries, September 11, 2017, https://ehtrust.org/wp-content/uploads/Scientist-5G-appeal-2017.pdf.

61. Ibid.

62. Camilla Rees, MBA, "EMF hygiene—How to Minimize Health Risks of Wireless Devices," *Holistic Primary Care,* June 9, 2011, https://holisticprimarycare.net/topics/environomics/emf-hygiene-how-to-minimize-health-risks-from-wireless-devices/.

63. Magda Havas is a professor of environmental and resource studies at Trent University in Peterboro, Ontario, Canada. She researches the biological effects of non-ionizing frequencies in the electromagnetic spectrum. This includes extremely low frequency (ELF) EMFs; intermediate frequencies (IF), commonly referred to as dirty electricity; radio frequency and microwave radiation (EMR); infrared radiation (IR); and light frequencies, including ultraviolet (UV) radiation. She has worked with human subjects and studied the effects of various frequencies

on plants, bees, farm animals, and microbes. For more information, see https://magdahavas.com.

64. "EWG Verified: A New Standard for Your Health," Environmental Working Group, https://www.ewg.org/ewgverified/about-the-mark.php, accessed June 2, 2021.

65. "Safe Drinking Water Act: Consumer Confidence Reports," US Environmental Protection Agency, September 25, 2020. https://www.epa.gov/ccr.

66. The author of *Detoxify or Die,* Sherry A. Rogers is board certified by the American Board of Environmental Medicine; a fellow of the American College of Allergy, Asthma and Immunology; and a fellow of the American College of Nutrition.

Chapter 21: A Wake Up Call for Us All

1. *Toxic—Heal Your Body from Mold Toxicity, Lyme Disease, Multiple Chemical Sensitivities, and Chronic Environmental Illness,* 306.

2. "Why Functional Medicine Matters: The Problem of Health Care: High Cost and Dependency," https://www.ifm.org/functional-medicine/why-functional-medicine-matters, accessed June 4, 2021.

3. C.K. Issak and Y.L. Siow, "The Evolution of Nutrition Research," *Canadian Journal of Physiology and Pharmacology.* 91(4) pp. 257-67, January 18, 2013, https://europepmc.org/article/med/23627837

4. Definition of "Nutrigenomics," *Nature.com,* https://www.nature.com/subjects/nutrigenomics, accessed June 4, 2021.

5. Marten H. Hofker, Jingyuan Fu, and Cisca Wijmenga, "The genome revolution and its role in understanding complex diseases," *ScienceDirect.com,* Volume 1842, Issue 10, October 2014, 1889-1895, https://www.sciencedirect.com/science/article/pii/S0925443914001306.

6. *The Mind-Gut Connection—How the Hidden Conversation Within Our Bodies Impacts Our Mood, Our Choices, and Our Overall Health,* 273.

7. Florence Williams is an American journalist and nonfiction author whose work focuses on the environment, health and science.

8. *Toxin Toxout—Getting Harmful Chemicals Out of Our Bodies and Our World,* book review by Evita Ochel for Evolving Wellness, May 23, 2014 (updated March 21, 2019), https://www.evolvingwellness.com/post/book-review-toxin-toxout.

9. Winston Churchill, "A Four-Year Plan for England," Post-War Councils on World Problems, broadcast from London over BBC, March 21, 1943, http://www.ibiblio.org/pha/policy/1943/1943-03-21a.html.

10. *Surviving Mold,* 40.

11. Ibid., 26.

12. *Toxic—Heal Your Body from Mold Toxicity, Lyme Disease, Multiple Chemical Sensitivities, and Chronic Environmental Illness,* 307.

Chapter 22: An Evolving Renaissance in Brain Wellness

1. *The End of Alzheimer's—The First Program to Prevent and Reverse Cognitive Decline,* 171-217.

2. Kat Toups, Ann Hathaway, Deborah Gordon, Henrianna Chung, Cyrus Raji, Alan Boyd, Benjamin D. Hill, Sharon Hausman-Cohen, Mouna Attarha, Won Jong Chwa, Michael Jarrett, and Dale E. Bredesen. "Precision Medicine Approach to Alzheimer's Disease: Successful Proof-of-Concept Trial," *MedRxiv* May 10, 2021. doi: https://doi.org/10.1101/2021.05.10.21256982; Statistics from the study noted on https://www.apollohealthco.com/clinical-trial-results-2021/

3. Dale E. Bredesen, MD, *The First Survivors of Alzheimer's* (New York, Penguin-Random House, 2021, 134).

4. Ibid., 18

5. TM Srinivasan, "Energy medicine," *International Journal of Yoga,* January 2010: 3(1), 1, https://pubmed.ncbi.nlm.nih.gov/20948893/.

6. Joanne DeLuca and Janine Lopiano are the co-founders of the future-forecasting consultancy, Sputnik Futures. For more information, see https://www.sputnikfutures.com/.

7. Beth *McGroarty with Joanne DeLuca and Janine Lopiano, co-founders, Sputnik Futures,* "Energy medicine gets serious," *2020 Global Wellness Trends,* https://www.globalwellnesssummit.com/2020-global-wellness-trends/energy-medicine-gets-serious/.

8. National Institute for Integrated Healthcare, https://niih.org/, accessed June 2, 2021.

9. "Photobiomodulation or low-level laser therapy."

10. Shang-Ru Tsai and Michael R. Hamblin, "Biological effects and medical applications of infrared radiation," *Journal of Photochemistry and Photobiology,* Volume 170, 197–207, May 2017, https://www.sciencedirect.com/science/article/abs/pii/S1011134416311691. You can find additional information in an article by Julio C. Rojas and F. Gonzalez-Lima, "Low-level light therapy of the eye and brain," *Eye and Brain,* Volume 2011, 49-67, October 17, 2011, https://www.dovepress.com/low-level-light-therapy-of-the-eye-and-brain-peer-reviewed-fulltext-article-EB.

11. Veterans Affairs Research Communications, "Can light therapy help the brain?" (April 2, 2015). *Science Daily,* April 2, 2015, https://www.sciencedaily.com/releases/2015/04/150402161648.htm.

12. Ibid.

13. "Introduction to Optogenetics," reviewed by Afsaneh Khetrapal, BSc, *News Medical /Life Sciences,* May 24, 2019, https://www.news-medical.net/life-sciences/Introduction-to-Optogenetics.aspx.

14. John E. Upledger, "Toxic Brain Injury (Encephalopathy)," *Massage Today,* Volume 04, Issue 07, July 2004, reprint appeared in International Alliance of Healthcare Educators, https://www.iahe.com/docs/articles/2852_001.pdf.

15. "Scientists discover previously unknown cleansing system in brain," Neuroscience News, August 15, 2012, https://neurosciencenews.com/glymphatic-system-cleansing-brain-glial-cells/. Also, see article by Michael Morgan, "Brain Toxins Be Gone! The Role of the Glymphatic System Revealed, *HuffPost,* August 31, 2017, https://www.iahe.com/docs/articles/brain-toxins-be-gone--the-role-of-the-glymphatic-system-revealed.pdf.

16. Michael Morgan, "Craniosacral Therapy is Being Explored as Treatment for Alzheimer's Disease," *Massage Magazine,* June 5, 2018, https://www.massagemag.com/craniosacral-treatment-for-alzheimers-89503/.

17. Erik L. Goldman, "Neuroacoustics: The Healing Power of Sound," *The Center for Neuroacoustic Research,* Volume 5, No. 3, Fall 2004, https://www.scientificsounds.com/library/neuroacoustics-the-healing-power-of-sound.

18. Ibid.

19. Lili Naghdi, Heidi Ahonen, Pasqualino Macario, and Lee Bartel, "The Effect of Low-Frequency Sound Stimulation on Patients with Fibromyalgia: A Clinical Study," *Pain Research & Management,* Volume 20, Article ID 375174, e21–e27, https://www.hindawi.com/journals/prm/2015/375174/.

20. Jason Alvarez, "New CRISPR Technology Offers Unrivaled Control of Epigenetic Inheritance," *University of California San Francisco Magazine,* April 15, 2021, https://www.ucsf.edu/news/2021/04/420306/new-crispr-technology-offers-unrivaled-control-epigenetic-inheritance.

21. Ariel Bleicher, "Technology will soon give us precise control over our brains and genes," *University of California San Francisco Magazine,* Winter 2020, https://www.ucsf.edu/magazine/control-brains-genes.

22. "Energy medicine gets serious."

Chapter 23: Managing the Collateral Chaos from Chronic Illness

1. "What is Long-Term Care (LTC) and Who Needs It?" U.S. Department of Health and Human Services, LongTermCare.gov, 2020, https://acl.gov/ltc.

Chapter 24: Caregiving and Care Issues

1. XRX Florida: Alzheimer's Disease and Related Dementias for Home Health: "Working with Families and Caregivers," AtrainEducation, https://www.atrainceu.com/content/5-working-families-and-caregivers, accessed June 3, 2021.

2. "2021 Alzheimer's Disease Facts and Figures."

3. "Help for Caregivers: Family Care Toolbox," *Caregiver Action Network,* https://caregiveraction.org/family-caregiver-toolbox, accessed June 3, 2021.

4. "2021 Alzheimer's Disease Facts and Figures."

5. "By 2030, All Baby Boomers Will Be Age 65 or Older: 2020 Census Will Help Policymakers Prepare for the Incoming Wave of Aging Boomers," United States Census Bureau, https://www.census.gov/library/stories/2019/12/by-2030-all-baby-boomers-will-be-age-65-or-older.html.

6. Max Ehrmann wrote this poem in 1927, but because he failed to copyright it at the appropriate time it became public domain. https://www.desiderata.com/desiderata.html.

Appendix A: Recognizing Neurotoxicity

1. "Positron Emissions Topography Scan: Overview." Mayo Clinic, August 25, 2020, https://www.mayoclinic.org/tests-procedures/pet-scan/about/pac-20385078.

2. What is Brain SPECT Imaging? Amen Clinics, http://www.amenclinics.com/approach/why-spect/, accessed June 4, 2021.

Appendix B: The Ticking Time Bomb of Lyme

1. Lorraine Johnson, "Lyme Disease Costs May Exceed $75 Billion Per Year," *LymeDisease.org,* https://www.lymedisease.org/members/lyme-times/special-issues/tick-borne-disease/lyme-disease-costs/, accessed February 17, 2021.

2. Kenneth Blum, Edward J. Modestino, Marcelo Febo, Bruce Steinberg, Thomas McLaughlin, Lyle Fried, David Baron, David Siwicki, and Rajendra D. Badgaiyan, "Lyme and dopaminergic function: Hypothesizing reduced reward deficiency symptomatology by regulating dopamine transmission," *Journal of Systems and Integrative Neuroscience,* 3(3), 10.15761/JSIN.1000163, May 2017, https://www.oatext.com/Lyme-and-dopaminergic-function-Hypothesizing-reduced-reward-deficiency-symptomatology-by-regulating-dopamine-transmission.php.

3. Lyme Disease: How many people get Lyme disease?" Centers for Disease Control and Prevention, https://www.cdc.gov/lyme/stats/humancases.html, accessed February 15, 2021.

Appendix C: The Forbidden Foods on an Amylose-Free Diet

1. "What is an Amylose Free Diet and Why Follow It?" moldfreemenu.com, https://moldfreemenu.com/can-a-low-amylose-diet-help-heal-mold-sickness/, accessed February 17, 2021.

2. Ibid., "CIRS Foods."

Appendix D: Common Symptoms of Lewy Body Dementia

1. "Symptoms," Lewy Body Dementia Association, www.lbda.org/symptoms/, accessed August 18, 2021.

Appendix E: Differences between Lewy Body Dementia and Alzheimer's Disease

1. "Is it Lewy Body Dementia or Something Else?" Lewy Body Dementia Association, https://www.lbda.org/is-it-lbd-or-something-else/, accessed July 7, 2021.

Appendix F: Functional Evaluation for Type 3 (Toxic) Alzheimer's Disease

1. Dale E. Bredesen, MD, "Inhalational Alzheimer's disease: an unrecognized—and treatable—epidemic," *Aging*, Volume 8, Issue 2, February 10, 2016, https://www.aging-us.com/article/100896/text.

Resources

Fortunately, there are now many articles, videos, podcasts, directories, and other resources available for further exploration related to toxicity, autoimmune disorders, brain diseases, functional medicine, and other health and wellness topics. Those listed provide a starting point for gathering vital information. Additionally, you will find an expansive array of materials featured on individual practitioners' websites for gaining additional wellness wisdom.

Check directory listings in some of the professional associations listed here for functional/integrative/naturopathic practitioners. Many practitioners now offer telemedicine services for your convenience and greater accessibility.

Alzheimer's Association: Provides information about dementia statistics, symptoms, stages, evaluation and treatment, caregiving, and many other concerns related to the disease. It also connects you to professionals and outlines support options. http://alz.org

Alzheimer's—The Science of Prevention **documentary**: A web-based documentary series hosted by neurologist, David Perlmutter, MD. The series features interviews with more than 20 recognized experts who explore the disease and what people can do to dramatically reduce their risk. https://drperlmutter.com

American Holistic Health Association: Impartial clearinghouse for finding wellness resources including a practitioner directory. https://ahha.org

Apollo Health: Dr. Dale Bredesen, Apollo's Chief Science Officer is at the forefront of research into Alzheimer's disease prevention and memory-loss reversal. The Bredesen Protocol offered through PreCODE (for prevention) and ReCODE (for reversal) features science-based prevention and recovery evaluation and treatment for brain health. https://apollohealthco.com

Autoimmune Association: Offering resources for education, increasing public awareness, research, and patient services regarding the wide range of autoimmune illnesses. https://autoimmune.com

Biotoxins: See listings for:
　　　　Lyme Disease Association
　　　　Mold Free Menu
　　　　MoldHelp.org
　　　　Neil Nathan, MD
　　　　Survivingmold.com
　　　　The Toxic Mold Summit

Center for Food Safety: With its mission to empower people, support farmers, and protect the earth from the harmful impacts of industrial agriculture, its advocacy work is devoted to protecting and promoting your right to both safe food and a health-sustaining environment. https://centerforfood-safety.org

Cognitive Health Centers: apply Dr. Bredesen's evidence-based protocols in the treatment and prevention of Alzheimer's disease, dementia and other cognitive decline issues. https://cognitivehealthcenters.com/

Environmental Working Group: Organized to protect our environmental health by changing industry standards. Its areas of focus include toxic chemicals, food, water, farming, agriculture, energy, family health, personal care, household, and consumer products as well as regional issues. http://ewg.org

Family Caregiver Alliance and the **National Center on Caregiving:** The mission of the FCA is to improve the quality of life for caregivers, for family caregivers, and the people who receive their care. It offers a wide range of topics related to caring for another and for those serving as caregivers. https://caregiver.org

The National Center on Caregiving also offers programs for family caregivers and resources for older or disabled adults living at home or in a residential facility. These are included in the same website listed above.

Food Revolution Network: Aims to empower individuals, build community, and transform food systems to support healthy people and a healthy planet. https://foodrevolution.org/

Foundation for Alternative and Integrative Health: FAIM's mission is to create a revolution in worldwide healthcare pursuing new frontiers in science and medicine to find cutting edge alternative and complimentary healthcare therapies. It features videos, podcasts, and articles on a wide range of health and wellness topics. https://faim.org

GreenMedInfo: "The Science of Natural Healing": An evidence-based natural health resource with more than 20,000 articles. https://greenmedinfo.com

Institute for Functional Medicine: Advancing the adoption of functional medicine practices for all. Includes a directory of member practitioners. Resources featuring functional medicine news and emerging research. https://ifm.org

Institute for Natural Medicine: a nonprofit organization partnered with naturopathic doctors who are focused on whole patient care, using diet, lifestyle and other ways to support the body's natural healing. Includes educational resources for consumers. https://naturemed.org

International Academy of Oral Medicine & Toxicology: a global network of dentists, health professionals, and scientists dedicated to protecting public health and the environment. Includes informative dental topics for consumers and a practitioner directory. https://iaomt.org

International Society for Environmentally Acquired Illness (ISEAI): is a non-profit medical society that aims to raise awareness of the environmental causes of inflammatory illnesses and to support the recovery of individuals affected by these illnesses through the integration of clinical practice, education, and research. https://iseai.org/

Lewy Body Dementia Association: dedicated to raising awareness of LBD, supporting people with LBD, their families, caregivers, and promoting scientific advances. https://lbda.org

Lyme Disease Association: Information regarding Lyme disease symptoms, Lyme disease treatments and other Lyme resources and educational materials for patients, medical professionals, researchers, educators, and policy makers. http://lymediseaseassociation.org

Mold: See listings under Biotoxins

MoldHelp.org: With its desire to increase awareness of the under-recognized illnesses caused by toxic mold, this organization is dedicated to offering information and support to people whose lives are impacted and often devastated by the effects of mold exposure: https://mold-help.org

Mold Free Menu: Dedicated to helping you create menus containing low amylose food choices for reducing inflammation in recovery from mold illness. https://moldfreemenu.com/

National Institute on Aging: Information on Alzheimer's Disease and related dementias, providing news, tips, and resources for caregivers and healthcare professionals. https://www.nia.nih.gov/health/alzheimers

Neil Nathan, MD: Specializing in treating patients whose environmental illnesses have made them especially sensitive and hard to treat: https://neilnathanmd.com

Preventive Medicine Research Institute: a non-profit, public institute dedicated to research, education and service demonstrating how lifestyle medicine can reverse, treat and prevent chronic disease.

The Renewal Point: Founded in 2003 by Dan Watts, MD, this integrative practice provides individualized care and treatment plans for patients around the world using state-of-the-art technologies and testing. By focusing on the four cornerstones of health—hormone balancing, nutritional health, physical conditioning, and toxin elimination—they help patients not only recover from major illness and disease, but also achieve optimal health and wellness. Following evidenced-based medicine and education, they combine the most reliable and effective therapies from traditional, metabolic, functional, and regenerative medicine. http://therenewalpoint.com

Safer Chemicals/Healthier Families: Advocates for strong chemical policies, working with businesses and organizations to phase out hazardous chemicals, and to educate the public to protect citizens from toxic chemicals. https://saferchemicals.org

SurvivingMold.com: A comprehensive resource regarding diagnosis, treatment, symptoms, remediation, educational resources, and physician network certified in the Shoemaker Protocol for biotoxin-related illnesses. https://survivingmold.com

The Toxic Mold Summit: a video series of interviews with functional and naturopathic practitioners hosted by Margaret Christensen, MD, featuring a wide range of topics related to mold toxicity, treatments, recovery, mold inspection and remediation. http://toxicmold.byhealthmeans.com

The Weston A. Price Foundation: WAPF provides information and scientific validation regarding food, nutrition, and health topics. It offers ideas for including nourishing traditional foods in your diet through wise choices and proper preparation techniques. http://westernaprice.org

Index

A

chemicals:

I

M

O

obesity:

    artificial sweeteners and, 127-128

    chronic inflammation and, 38, 233

    cognitive decline and, 141, 183

    glyphosate and, 125

    gut issues and, 134

    hormonal imbalances and, 127-128

    toxicity and, 32, 113, 123

O'Bryan, Dr. Tom, 118

off-gassing of toxins, 111

olive oil, 176, 178

optic neuritis, 87

optogenetics, 201

organic foods, 124, 177-180

oxidative stress, 161-162; 174-179

oxybenzone, 116

ozone therapy, 172

P

PAI-1, 32

pain:

    abdominal, 139

    Bell's Palsy and, 87

    management, 42-44, 179, 183-184, 203

    nerve, 27, 162, 142, 162

    Rick's description, 13, 19-20, 42-44, 46, 217-218, 222

    symptom of toxicity and, v, 26-28, 31-34, 72, 78, 121, 145, 229, 232

    toxic tort cases, 111-112

pancreas, 130, 181

parabens, 116

survivingmold.com, 30, 278

sweat, 15, 172

T

tau, 105, 129, 173, 176, 183

Teflon, 116, 187

temperature regulation, 19-20, 30, 32-33, 235

Thompson, Dr. Jeffrey, 203

thyroid, 7, 13, 115, 148, 243

   See also Hashimoto thyroiditis

TNF alpha (tumor necrosis factor alpha), 128-129, 246

toluene, 111, 116-117

tomatoes, 137, 179

toxic encephalopathy. *See* encephalopathy

toxins:

  off-gassing of, 111

  Smart Choices in Today's Toxic Times, 170-190

  See also amalgam fillings; biotoxins; chemicals; EMFs; detoxification; GMOs; heavy metals; Lyme disease; mold

Toxin-Toxout, 164,194

trans fats, 180, 234

tremor(s), v, viii, 5, 13, 19, 33, 46, 78, 91, 146, 235

triclosan, 116-117

Trojanowski, Dr. John, 105

trusts, 208

turmeric, 165, 171, 179

Type 3 (toxic) Alzheimer's disease:

  biochemical markers, 103-106, 238-240

  characteristics of, 238-240

  similar characteristics to LBD, 103-106

Western Blot test, 35, 71, 75

wi-fi exposure, 187-188

Williams, Florence, 193

Williams, Robin, v, 17

wills, 207-208

X

xylene, 111

Z

zeolite, 172

zinc, 138, 239, 243